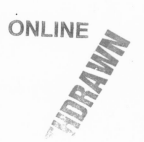

THE
KNEE
SOURCEBOOK

—

Marc Darrow, M.D., J.D.

Contemporary Books

Chicago   New York   San Francisco   Lisbon   London   Madrid   Mexico City
Milan   New Delhi   San Juan   Seoul   Singapore   Sydney   Toronto

Library of Congress Cataloging-in-Publication Data

Darrow, Marc, M.D.
    The knee sourcebook / by Marc Darrow.
      p.   cm.
    Includes bibliographical references and index.
    ISBN 0-7373-0544-4 (alk. paper)
    1. Knee—Wounds and injuries.   2. Knee—Diseases.   I. Title.

    RD561.D375   2001
    617.5'82—dc21   2001037282

Contemporary Books

*A Division of The **McGraw·Hill** Companies*

1 2 3 4 5 6 7 8 9 0   AGM/AGM   0 9 8 7 6 5 4 3 2 1

ISBN 0-7373-0544-4

This book was set in Minion and Helvetica Neustedt by Robert S. Tinnon Design
Printed and bound by Quebecor Martinsburg

Cover design by Cheryl Carrington
Interior design by Robert S. Tinnon

McGraw-Hill books are available at special quantity discounts to use as premiums and sales promotions, or for use in corporate training programs. For more information, please write to the Director of Special Sales, Professional Publishing, McGraw-Hill, Two Penn Plaza, New York, NY 10121-2298. Or contact your local bookstore.

This book is printed on acid-free paper.

Contents

Foreword

I am honored to write the foreword to *The Knee Sourcebook* by Dr. Marc Darrow. Marc's straightforward, understandable writing style will help patients, general practitioners, chiropractors, physical therapists, and naturopathic health care workers to understand the subtle complexities of one of the most commonly injured joints. He clearly defines the anatomy of the knee, describes common problems facing all of us, and brings a fresh perspective to treatment alternatives.

Marc infuses the book with his personal philosophy of care and demonstrates how a health care provider should treat and communicate with his patients. I have been fortunate enough to know Marc both professionally and personally for many years. In his practice he uses a multidisciplinary approach combined with a New Age philosophy, and a personal interest in each patient's individual needs. Marc's approach marries many aspects of traditional medicine, the latest options in regimen, and newer holistic and alternative medicine therapies.

As an orthopedic surgeon specializing in sports medicine and arthroscopic surgery, I've had the opportunity and privilege to treat some of the top national, international, and professional athletes in the world. I have long recognized that rehabilitative medicine is truly the key to a successful surgical outcome. Commonly, therapy starts with exercises to regain range of motion and methods to relieve pain, reduce swelling, and decrease inflammation. The next phase of rehabilitation is a program to strengthen the knee stabilizers. At this point, most therapies stop. Dr. Darrow and I advocate continuing an aggressive therapy program to regain proprioception (the innate ability of the body to know where the limb is in space) and motor retraining to regain quickness and muscle memory. Late rehabilitation also includes sport-specific drills.

Knee surgery and rehabilitation have undergone phenomenal changes and progress over the last twenty-five years. Basic scientific research, new surgical techniques, and advances in equipment have allowed the orthopedic surgeon to offer patients a wider array of treatment options both surgically and nonsurgically than ever before.

Twenty-five years ago a patient with a torn meniscus (cartilage) would require a formal open knee operation (arthrotomy) and removal of the entire meniscal cartilage. The patient usually spent a week in the hospital, was put in a cast for six weeks, and could expect a year of painful rehabilitation. Late arthritic change of the knee was predictable, and, much later, knee replacement surgery would be necessary.

Better ways to manage the damaged knee came, like most advances in medicine, through serendipity. A Japanese gynecologist, Dr. Masaki Watanabe, developed a surgical telescope to use in the abdomen. As this "scope" was made smaller and more refined, and the field of fiber optics (an offshoot of the space and telecommunication programs) advanced, the arthroscope was born. In the late 1970s an orthopedic surgeon could for the first time look into the knee and make a firm diagnosis of whether a meniscus was torn. Another four or five years passed until instrumentation was perfected to allow doctors to perform surgery "through the scope." True operative arthroscopy also relied on advances in video technology. Once reliable, sterilizable cameras and lens optics were perfected, surgeons no longer had to have their eye directly on the scope to visualize the knee. The use of video enhanced the sterility of the procedure and opened the door to a wider variety of surgical procedures, including partial removal of the meniscus, removal of loose bodies, and eventually anterior cruciate ligament reconstruction.

By the mid-1980s the preferred way of managing a meniscal injury of the knee was outpatient arthroscopic surgery and removal of only the torn portion of the meniscus. This is especially important today, because the baby boomers are playing more sports, competing harder and longer, and sustaining a high number of knee injuries later in life. Procedures once reserved for the elite young athlete are now commonplace for the weekend warrior and even the couch potato.

I find it interesting that, in the old days of ligament reconstructions and immobilizing patients in casts for months, often the "noncompliant patient" had the best results. The active patients who became frustrated and removed their own casts would start moving their knee even though it was "against medical advice." Today, I don't place patients in a cast at all, and I start motion in the recovery room with a constant passive motion machine. I routinely expect patients to obtain full extension and 110 to 125 degrees of flexion within two weeks. Crutches are usually necessary for only a week, and weight-bearing is permitted immediately.

What's on the horizon to help the competing athlete, the aging athlete, or the person with a degenerative knee? Therapies run the gamut from injectable solutions that help nourish, strengthen, and rebuild articular cartilage to unicompartmental and tricompartmental total knee replacements. Recent work has been done to grow articular (surface) cartilage in the laboratory and place it in the knee to repair local arthritic conditions. Tissue from cadavers is used for knee ligament and meniscal replacements, prolotherapy is used for strengthening collagen, and spacers are used to realign degenerative knees.

Working closely with Marc Darrow, I have sought and shared opinions, advice, and information about new therapies. But I've learned more from Marc than just medicine or science. His true love of medicine and his heartfelt and sincere caring for his patients have reinstilled in me a passion for medicine. Marc sets a high standard, practicing the art of medicine with sensitivity and caring, based on a foundation of spirituality and integrity. His philosophy—joy of living and joy of giving—permeates the office and flows from doctor to patient and patient to doctor.

GARY BRAZINA, M.D.

Acknowledgments

I have been fortunate to have many wonderful teachers in my life. Their love has kept me focused to become all that I am. Among the most important have been my parents and my mentor, John-Roger. They supported me through my trials by fire. John-Roger delivered me from my questing hippie years in Berkeley, California, to wondrous careers in law and medicine.

Were it not for my wife, Michelle, and her little clones, Jensen, Brittany, and Jordan, I would not have the joy and focus that allow me the sanity to carry on with my work. Benjy and Jason continually send me the light.

Together with Dr. Jason Kelberman, Dr. William Bergman, Dr. Frank Kaden, Dr. Gary Brazena, and our energetic team, we will continue to deliver the most loving form of medical healing available.

I am blessed to have all of you in my life.

Introduction

My earliest memories involve the romance of medicine. As a young boy, I hiked in the Indiana sand dunes with my grandfather Edda, a high-minded doctor. He constantly prodded me with the wisdom of the ages and the virtues of the early philosophers.

There was nothing else I wanted to do but heal.

Modern medicine has taken a diversion from the days of Edda when surgery was not a real option. Today most people want a quick fix so they can return to their cyberspace lifestyle. My experience as a doctor is that the quick fix may later turn into an unexpected chronic problem.

My hope is that this book will start you on a path back to the roots of medicine that Edda believed in: that healing is a natural process that takes initiative by the patient.

Be sure to explore the many avenues of healing available to you. With the advent of the information age and the Internet, you can be quickly educated. It is certainly worth your time to find the most natural way to heal yourself. Above all, find a loving environment in which to heal.

I am in love with medicine, and yet the term *doctor* has, in part, a negative connotation for me. As a medical student in Hawaii, when patients called me Dr. Darrow, I would reply that I am not a doctor but a medical student. They would respond, "Yes, Dr. Darrow." I did not wish to be held in the honor of my respected teachers without having earned the right.

Throughout the past several years, I have become disillusioned with the pedestal on which society has placed doctors. Our job as doctors is to minister to others, not to treat patients as a "diagnosis." Every one of us has an individual spiritual heart, needing love and personal recognition. We are neither recipes in a cookbook, nor automobiles that can be tuned up by mechanical device.

Very few of us fit the mold of modern algorithmic medicine taught in medical school and practiced in hospitals. The greatest fault of our medical teaching system is that the major emphasis is placed on critical-care hospital-based medicine, while the majority of patients are seen in an outpatient setting in doctor's offices. What happened to teaching doctors to deal with the problems of patients who are not critically ill? Why is it that during four years of medical school we had only one lecture on nutrition?

On the positive side, many medical schools are being forced by student demand to give courses on alternative medicine. Strangely, what we call *alternative medicine* has been around since the beginning of time. Nevertheless, while alternative medicine is demanded by patients who have found failure in the current medical model, it is still shunned by the majority of doctors who, unfortunately, do not know of its merits. Why? Medicine is run by a referral system. If a doctor does not follow the "party line," other doctors will be afraid to send him or her patients. No doctor wishes to be ostracized by his or her peers in this tight-knit community.

When a patient walks into my office and calls me Dr. Darrow, I respond, "Please, call me Marc." I immediately notice the person relax, knowing it will be a new experience, being on the same level with his doctor. Instead of just listening to their problems, I also share my own trials and tribulations, and I think this reflects my ordinariness. This allows a person to be my friend and share with me on a deep and esoteric level. Once that common ground is met, the concept of healing from within can be presented.

According to the American Academy of Orthopaedic Surgeons, more than six million people seek medical care each year for a knee problem. Knee pain is most often the result of repetitive wear (such as what occurs in osteoarthritis), trauma (such as a blow to the knee), or sudden movements that strain the knee beyond its normal range of motion (such as those that occur in tennis, skiing, skating, household falls, etc.). Unfortunately, the knee is the most commonly injured joint, accounting for 26 percent of all orthopedic visits.

Whether you are in the best shape of your life, a weekend athlete, or now suffering trauma and pain caused by a lifetime of common wear and tear—I have written this sourcebook for you. In this book, I will discuss:

- How the knee is designed and how it functions.
- Common knee injuries such as tears and sprains of the ligaments, tendons, cartilage, meniscus, and bones forming the joint.
- Strengthening exercises that can help prevent injury.
- Diseases and syndromes of the knee, including tendinitis (inflammation of a tendon), iliotibial band syndrome (inflammation caused by friction and long-term overuse), and osteochondritis dissecans (a degeneration of the blood supply to the bone).
- Related conditions such as osteoarthritis that cause knee pain.
- Alternative therapies, such as magnetic resonance and collagen rejuvenating prolotherapy.

Chapter One

The Functioning Knee

It's a beautiful Sunday afternoon. One minute you're racing your pal down the driveway to the basketball hoop, leaping for the shot of a lifetime; the next you're dropping to the asphalt, betrayed by a knee that doesn't share your NBA fantasies. As you hobble to the living room, your only consolation is that there's a football game on TV. It isn't long before the crowd is on its feet—not because of a spectacular play but because a star forward just got sacked, and he's now in the same place you are: groaning in pain and wondering why that knee of his has let him down.

The truth is, the knee lasts a lot longer—and works a lot better—than most of us deserve. It suffers regular stress from our everyday life habits: pounding runs on pavement; extra pounds it's not meant to carry; excessive movement due to ligament, tendon, and joint capsule injuries; muscle atrophy because of inactivity; or tension and tendon shortening induced by designer high heels. It's amazing the knee can support us at all.

Support most of us it does, however, through a remarkable system of joints and cartilage; muscles, ligaments, and tendons; and the fibrous collagen that holds it all together. However, it often does not support us with ease, and in extreme cases it can no longer support us at all. The old saying is true: "The knees are the first to go."

Clearly, many of us have trouble with our knees at some point in our lives. To minimize your own risk and understand how to protect the knee from injury—or promote healing once it's been pushed to the point of straining or tearing—you need to have a clear comprehension of how the knee works.

HOW THE KNEE WORKS (AND DOESN'T)

The skeletal structure has two primary types of joints—the ball joint, exemplified by the shoulder, which allows free rotation (a freedom that comes with its own set of problems and injuries, by the way); and the hinge joint, illustrated by the knee, which operates primarily in a single plane (bent to straight) with only a slight rotational or pivoting motion. This restriction of movement is what makes the knee so vulnerable to traumatic injury. Additionally, the knee is regularly subjected to the stress of both supporting body weight and absorbing shock from intermittent impacts such as jumping, walking, and running. Over time these stresses cause a loosening of the connective ligaments, the tendons, and the joint capsule that holds the knee together. Along with a wearing away of cushioning cartilage and collagen, this loosening leads to the pain and dysfunction of bone meeting bone. At its worst, this condition manifests as arthritis.

ANATOMY OF THE KNEE

The knee is made up of bones, ligaments, tendons, cartilage, and a joint capsule, all of which are composed of collagen. Ligaments connect bone to bone. Tendons attach muscle to bone. Cartilage is the smooth, fibrous connective tissue covering bones that allows easy, gliding movement.

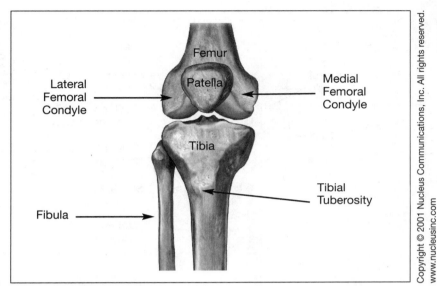

Within the figure:
Femur
Patella
Lateral Femoral Condyle
Medial Femoral Condyle
Tibia
Tibial Tuberosity
Fibula

Figure 1.1: Bones of the Knee

Collagen is the fibrous protein constituent of connective tissue present throughout the body. As we age, the most obvious sign of collagen breakdown is in the face, where it leads to the sagging that keeps plastic surgeons in business. Less obviously, however, collagen breaks down throughout the body and contributes to a variety of age-related injuries and conditions. These keep orthopedic surgeons in business. However, treatments and methods other than surgery may do a better job of preserving and rejuvenating the knee (see chapters 5 to 8).

The knee joint is a link between the thighbone—the femur—and the two bones of the lower leg—the tibia (large and on the inside) and the fibula (small and on the outside). The attaching ligaments on the outer surfaces of the knee are the medial collateral ligament (connecting the tibia to the femur) and the lateral collateral ligament (connecting the fibula to the femur). The patellar tendon

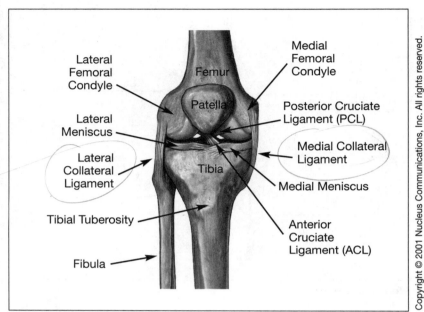

Lateral
Femoral
Condyle

Femur

Medial
Femoral
Condyle

Patella

Lateral
Meniscus

Posterior Cruciate
Ligament (PCL)

Medial Collateral
Ligament

Lateral
Collateral
Ligament

Tibia

Medial Meniscus

Tibial Tuberosity

Anterior
Cruciate
Ligament (ACL)

Fibula

Figure 1.2: Knee Bones with Ligaments

attaches the quadriceps muscles of the thigh to the tibia, enabling extension of the knee. Inside the knee joint, two ligaments stretch between the femur and tibia—the anterior cruciate ligament and, behind it, the posterior cruciate ligament. Covering the ends of the bones is articular cartilage, which provides a smooth surface to facilitate motion. *Articular* cartilage is so named because when bones move against each other, they are said to *articulate*. In the knee, articular cartilage covers the end of the femur, the top of the tibia, and the back of the patella (the kneecap). In the middle of the knee joint are the menisci, which are collagenous disc-shaped cushions that act as shock absorbers.

Unlike a ball joint, such as the hip, which sits in a deep pocket (the acetabulum of the pelvis), the knee doesn't have much protection from trauma and stress. It is designed to move mostly in one

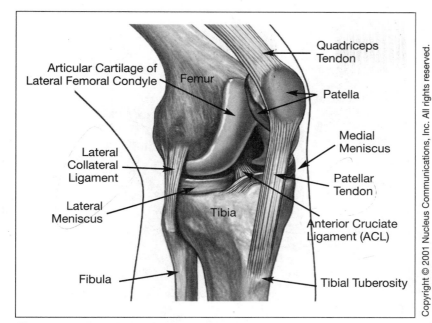

Figure 1.3: Anterior Lateral View of the Knee

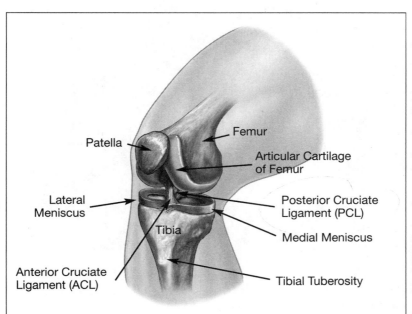

Figure 1.4: Anterior Medial View of the Knee

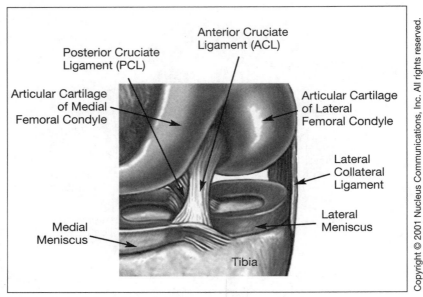

Figure 1.5: Frontal View of the Knee

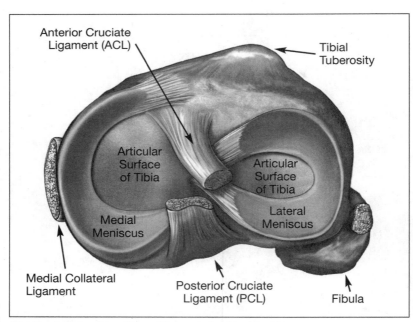

Figure 1.6: Looking Down Through the Healthy Knee

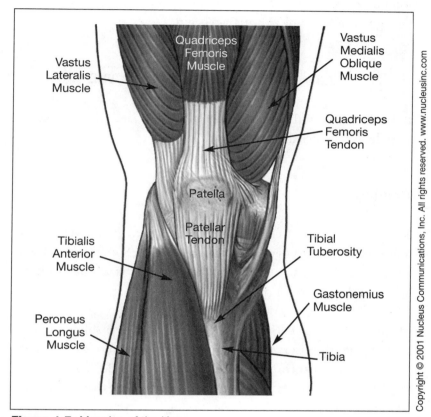

Vastus Lateralis Muscle

Quadriceps Femoris Muscle

Vastus Medialis Oblique Muscle

Quadriceps Femoris Tendon

Patella

Patellar Tendon

Tibialis Anterior Muscle

Tibial Tuberosity

Peroneus Longus Muscle

Gastonemius Muscle

Tibia

Figure 1.7: Muscles of the Knee

plane like a hinge. Because of this inherent limitation of movement, strong knee ligaments are extremely important for knee health.

Side-to-side stresses are controlled by the medial and lateral collateral ligaments; front-to-back motion is handled by the anterior and posterior cruciate ligaments, which ensure that the tibia doesn't slide backward or forward in relation to the femur. When these ligaments become lax, or are torn, bone movement may become excessive and damaging, and painful arthritis can begin.

DAILY FUNCTIONING OF THE KNEE

To further explain the functioning of the knee, let's focus on common daily activities that affect it.

Walking

No movement or exercise is easier on the knees than a well-paced, well-executed walk in good, comfortable shoes. Some factors, however, can make this most natural of motions hazardous to knee health, and I discuss those next.

Irregular Gait Gait is simply the way in which a person walks. In a perfect gait cycle, the pushing off and landing motions of the heel and toe are in balance, contributing to an even stride. Many people, however, unconsciously favor the heel or toe when they walk, contributing to an uneven and uncomfortable gait cycle.

Plantar flexion, favoring the toe, occurs when the foot is angled down at the ankle from heel to toes (at its most extreme, walking on tiptoe). This causes the knee to hyperextend (literally straighten too far), putting extreme pressure on the joint itself as well as its individual anatomical parts. The tendons, ligaments, and joint capsule are stretched so that they move out of place, resulting in a sprain or strain.

Dorsiflexion, favoring the heel, occurs when the foot is angled up from the ankle (at its most extreme, walking on the heels alone) so that the person falls forward, straining the quadriceps (thigh) muscles. Excess dorsiflexion keeps the quadriceps contracted in order to keep the individual from falling over and inhibits normal straightening of the knee.

Both of these gait deviations are commonly seen in people who have had a stroke, brain injury, or spinal cord injury and in children with cerebral palsy.

Shoes The common shoe offender to knee health is, of course, high heels. Their negative impact is compound. First, they position the foot so that its usefulness as a shock absorber is greatly diminished. This problem is exacerbated by the fact that the shoes themselves are often thin-soled and unpadded, offering no cushion between the foot and the pavement. Second, they create stress for the knee by causing prolonged muscle contraction and fatigue. Third, over the long haul, constant wearing of high heels can create a permanent tightening and shortening of the Achilles tendons, so that any shoes other than high heels become difficult and painful to wear.

Another source of problems is worn-out or improperly fitted athletic shoes. Designed to compensate for the impact caused by running, jogging, or jumping, shoes that become worn down create problems in two ways. First, a reduction in the cushion increases the impact on the knees. Second, soles worn down on their sides, heel, or toe may magnify the slight imperfection in gait that caused uneven wear in the first place. A shoe that fits poorly may cause poor toe-off (the beginning of a step) or excess muscle strain.

Jogging and Running

Jogging and running have benefits for both body and mind. Great calorie burners, they also clear your mind and renew your spirit, offering the much vaunted "runner's high." They can, however, take a real toll on the knees unless you take precautions. As discussed in the preceding section, good shoes are a must, and you should re-place them regularly if you are a frequent or long-distance runner. Carefully consider your running surface—a dirt track is better than a concrete one, and flat or uphill running is preferable to downhill. Most runners do pay attention to these factors.

Another predictor of potential knee problems as a runner is your physical build. *Q angle* (quadriceps angle) is measured by drawing a line from your anterior iliac spine (the bump on your pelvis above and in front of your hip joint) to the center of your kneecap, and a second line from your kneecap to the tibial tuberosity (the little bump at the top of the tibia where the patellar tendon attaches to your tibia).

A wide Q angle would be more than 15 degrees and might be found on extremely broad-hipped women. Such an angle may increase the likelihood of "runner's knee" (patellofemoral syndrome), because it predisposes a person to run with the knees pushed inward (knock-kneed). The resultant strain loosens the patellar tendon and its col-lagenous attachments and weakens their hold on the patella. The patella may then move off its track on the femur, resulting in pain and inflammation. A wide Q angle does not always cause pain and is not a reason to stop running, however; its effects can be adjusted by the use of orthotics or braces (these devices are discussed in chapter 7).

Squatting

In some cultures squatting is the preferred method of sitting and is practically an art form. People in those cultures can sustain the pos-ture for lengthy periods of time—astonishing to the average Ameri-can. Squatting is sometimes advocated for pregnant women as a way to ease the eventual difficulties of labor. When regular squatting is practiced from childhood, the knee suffers no ill effects. However, if you use this motion only occasionally—or incorporate it suddenly into your daily routine—it can cause problems. Certainly you may occasionally squat to pick up an errant sock or a sleeping child from the floor. Mostly, though, squatting in this country occurs during exercise.

A well-executed squat is an excellent muscle-toner and muscle-stabilizer, but a poorly executed one can create problems. Deep knee bends to a squatting position—once the cornerstone of military-inspired exercise regimes—have now been determined to do more harm than good by jamming the patella into the femur, and subluxing (partially dislocating) the femur from the tibia—in this case, slipping the femur over the tibia, outside its normal anatomical placement. Squatting may increase the forces on the knee joint up to eight times body weight.

Stair Climbing

Once used primarily by athletes in training, stair climbing has become popular with exercisers who take step classes in gyms and with aerobic enthusiasts who use the outdoor stairs at beaches, hills, and high school or college stadiums. A lot of them end up limping into the doctor's office with knees that just can't take the strain.

With stair climbing, the knee moves quite a bit and is under a great deal of pressure. The more the knee is flexed, the tighter the patellar tendon is stretched, pushing on the patella. When the tendon stretches out, the area where it attaches becomes inflamed, and tracking of the patella goes off course. It drifts, slips, and tilts, resulting in patellofemoral syndrome (runner's knee) or, in more extreme cases, chondromalacia patellae (wearing out of the cartilage on the back of the patella). Extreme wear and tear on the cartilage and menisci (the cushioning discs between the femur and the tibia), over time, roughen the glassy cartilage surface and decrease the protection it and the menisci offer. Eventually, bone may meet bone, causing painful arthritis.

Stair climbing may increase the force of the patella on the femur up to four times body weight. To help keep the exercise as safe for your knees as it is good for your metabolism and cardiac function, take care to give your knees a rest (don't do the same exercise two days in a row), alternate stair climbing with other types of exercise, reduce your speed while climbing, and pay immediate heed when your knees start to ache or swell.

Jumping

It's hard not to feel a twinge of envy when you watch your favorite six-year-old leap off the furniture, knowing the only damage she's likely to cause is to Mom's favorite breakable. As we get older, the impact of jumping is likely to have far more painful consequences than paying for repairs out of our allowance money. The harsh impact, combined with the potential for twisting and tearing, makes jumping a risky business indeed. Still, some of us can't resist. We rise into the air on driveway basketball courts and in funk-music-driven aerobics classes. Sometimes we land easily, sometimes we don't.

When you jump, even a good landing may compromise your knee joint. Those strong quadriceps muscles contract on landing and pull hard at the patellar tendon's insertion on the tibial tuberosity (the little bump at the top of the tibia). This may cause jumper's knee (inflammation of the patellar tendon). Of course, if you land off your intended, balanced course, you will strain all elements of your knee joint. The correct shoes and corrective knee bands can reduce knee injury when jumping.

LIFESTYLE AND THE KNEE

Two major contributors to knee health (or lack of it) affect us in most other areas of our health as well: excess weight and inactivity.

Weight

It isn't hard to imagine the effect excess weight has on your knees. Like a house, you have a frame designed to carry a certain amount of weight, and if you overload that frame it will begin to crumble under the load. The knee endures a great deal of punishment when overburdened, straining to carry far more than it was designed to. Everything is affected—cartilage may diminish; ligaments and tendons may stretch, wear out, and tear. While some treatments may give short-term relief, as long as the excess weight is there, the knee is inhibited from healing and may continue to deteriorate.

If excess weight is a problem for you, a low-carbohydrate diet works very effectively, not only to lose weight but also to lower blood pressure, lower blood glucose, lower cholesterol, and relieve heartburn, gas, and bloating.

Inactivity

The damage to your knees from inactivity is not immediately obvious, but it is a very real problem. It affects all aspects of the knee— muscles, tendons, ligaments, cartilage, bones, and collagen. Muscles atrophy extremely quickly—immobilized muscles (such as those in a cast) atrophy 28 percent in the first week. They weaken and become lax. Over time, inactivity weakens muscles the same way, so that they afford the knee less and less protection.

Cartilage in the knee is mostly avascular (that is, not fed by a blood supply). Instead, cartilage receives its nourishment through osmosis and pressure. Movement is what nourishes the cartilage. Without it, the knee is essentially "starved." The resultant loss of cartilage leads to the pain of bone on bone and degenerative conditions such as arthritis.

The contraction of muscle on bone also nourishes the bone—stimulating the osteoblasts, the cells that produce bone and make it dense. Dense bones minimize the chance of fracture.

Inactivity also starves the tendons, ligaments, and connective collagen, because motion is what forces blood supply to bring nutrients to these tissues. Without adequate blood supply, they tighten, stiffen, and contract, lessening their ability to cushion and protect.

WOMEN AND KNEE INJURIES

A number of recent studies have addressed a growing concern: Women are experiencing a far greater number of knee injuries than ever before and proportionally more than men incur. In fact, according to the National Collegiate Athletic Association, female athletes between the ages of nineteen and twenty-five are an astounding three to four times more likely to suffer an ACL injury than their male counterparts.

Why the increase in injury? Because more women of all ages are actively and aggressively participating in sports— both professionally and recreationally—than ever before.

Why are women more susceptible to injury? The answer to that is far less definitive, but researchers are finding clues—both physiological and cultural—that suggest ways in which women may protect themselves, until we can answer the question fully.

Training

Observations of female athletes reveal two primary differences between the sexes: Females tend to land from a jump on flat feet, while men tend to land on their toes; and women rely far more heavily on their quadriceps muscles (the muscles in the front of the thigh) than men do. In fact, when tested, female athletes' hamstring muscles (the muscles in back of the thigh) had merely 45 to 55 percent of the strength of their quadriceps. To perform safely as well as efficiently, hamstring strength should be 60 to 70 percent of quadriceps strength. Correcting the deficiency is simply a matter of training. Although patterns are changing, women have generally not been exposed to sports and weight training at the early ages that men have, and this lack of preconditioning may lead to later injury. Strength training, lunges, and drilling jumps with the proper toe-first landing may reduce a female athlete's injury rate to the same as a male's.

Body Structure

The quadriceps angle (Q angle), measured from the knee to the hip, is a factor in knee injuries. The greater Q angle of wide-hipped women may put them at risk for injury. This in no way precludes activity, but it increases the importance of prevention and strength training.

Hormone Levels

Although no researcher has found the reason for it, women's increased estrogen levels do seem to contribute to injury. The extra estrogen that women have might cause loose ligaments as it does during pregnancy to allow the baby to pass through the small birth canal. A 1998 University of Michigan study of female athletes, published in the *American Journal of Sports Medicine,* found that the greatest number of injuries occurred when estrogen levels were highest. Awareness may be the best prevention—extra concentration and focus on proper form during ovulation and even more during pregnancy could make the difference between being able to play and suffering an injury that keeps you warming the bench.

The Michigan study revealed a couple of other interesting facts: Sixty-one percent of female athletes' injuries occurred during a game, as opposed to training or practice; of those, 64 percent occurred in the first 30 minutes of play. One factor that didn't play a role in knee injuries was shoes—neither age nor brand seemed to make a difference when it came to protecting the female athlete.

OLDER ADULTS AND KNEE INJURIES

One common refrain among elderly people is: "I'm falling apart!" It sounds funny, but the fact is, it's true. Ligaments, tendons, and collagenous attachments loosen through time. Like a rubber band, they stretch, wear out, and lose shape. You see the outward effects and feel the painful inward ones—your body just can't seem to do what it once did.

The most common knee problems for older adults are pain and immobility related to osteoarthritis. Reduced bone mass from osteoporosis makes postmenopausal women more susceptible to injury. Weight-bearing exercise has been proved not only to reduce the risk of fracture but also to reduce pain for many osteoarthritis and osteoporosis sufferers.

How prevalent is knee pain in the older population? In a University of Michigan study, 48 percent of participants revealed ongoing pain in their backs and knees. A study conducted at Wake Forest University in Winston-Salem, North Carolina, and the University of Tennessee in Memphis, by Dr. Walter Ettinger and his colleagues (published in the *Journal of the American Medical Association* in 1997) showed that exercise may help. The researchers compared three groups of patients age sixty or older. The first did weight-bearing exercises, the second engaged in regular walking, and the third received only verbal instruction in health issues. After eighteen months of participation, those who exercised regularly—whether with weight-bearing activities or walking—experienced increased mobility and decreased pain.

Another problem for seniors is reduced ability to maintain balance. To improve balance, as well as strength and flexibility, many seniors are turning to the ancient Chinese art of tai chi chuan. The movements performed in tai chi are focused, slow, and precise, and they offer a number of benefits for seniors. To find a class nearby, check out www.thetaichisite.com.

Seniors, and others, who are concerned about their ability to exercise after knee-replacement surgery should be heartened by the findings published in 2000 by Swiss researcher Markus S. Kuster and his colleagues, who evaluated the compressive forces generated on the prosthetic (artificial) knee by four kinds of exercise: cycling, jogging, easy walking, and mountain hiking. The researchers evaluated three types of tibial inlays (a part of the prosthesis)—flat inlays, curved inlays, and inlays with mobile bearings—to determine the point at which the prosthetic joint became overloaded (the polyethylene became deformed) during the exercise.

Both cycling and easy walking were easily sustained without damage to the prosthetic joint. Jogging was, not surprisingly, the most damaging to the knee. Hiking offered mixed results—uphill climbing was not a problem, but sustained downhill hikes created undue pressure on the knee joint. The addition of a weighty backpack also created problems in the knee joint.

The final result is that a healthy recipient of a knee replacement can participate in all but the most jarring exercises. Hiking is possible, provided you plan a route without sustained downhill treks and avoid long hikes that require you to carry a lot of supplies in a heavy pack. Long walks and cycling trips are quite feasible. You may not be playing a lot of pickup basketball, but you can maintain a healthy, active lifestyle.

Exercise, of course, helps control excess weight, which is a major contributor to knee injuries and chronic pain. If you are older, female, and overweight, you are in a high-risk category for knee problems. Every step you take, and every pound you lose, can create a healthier, happier life.

The bad news is that you can't stop the aging process, but the good news is that you can inhibit it. Strength training, good nutrition, noticing and dealing with problems when they start—all of these will allow you to enjoy the benefits of aging (such as wisdom, more free time, and perhaps financial security) while avoiding the injuries that can occur if you pretend you're still fifteen until your knee collapses and you're forced to admit you're not.

Now that you have a general understanding of knee function, you can learn about knee injuries—how to determine the type of injury you've sustained and immediate steps to take so that you don't make it worse.

Chapter Two

Knee Injuries

One of the most difficult concepts to impart to an athlete is Einstein's definition of *crazy*: doing the same thing over and over and expecting different results. Athletes want to keep doing their sport with the same intensity in the same way. Their method of performance is to do the same thing over and over, and injury is the result. When an athlete visits a doctor, his expectation is that the doctor will create a magical healing so that the athlete can continue to repeat exactly what caused the injury. A great sage once said, "When you are sick and tired of being sick and tired, you'll change."

Knee injuries generally fall into one of two categories:

1. Traumatic: a sudden injury caused by either exterior impact (such as a football tackle) or an unintended twisting or hyperextension of the knee (such as a skiing fall).
2. Repetitive: problems such as "runner's knee" (patellofemoral syndrome) or iliotibial band syndrome that are created over time by doing a damaging motion again and again.

In addition, knees may suffer from pathological conditions (those that seem to be genetically predetermined or related to a disease). Some conditions, such as osteoarthritis, may result from a combination of genetics and traumatic or repetitive injury.

In this chapter we'll address the symptoms of traumatic and repetitive knee injuries and immediate steps to take so that you don't worsen your condition before it can be fully diagnosed medically and treated properly. Chapter 3 looks at pathological knee conditions, and chapter 4 discusses diagnosis of the injured knee.

TRAUMATIC INJURIES

Anyone who has suffered a traumatic knee injury knows how painful, and how frightening, it can be. The most common traumatic knee injuries are described in the sections that follow.

Anterior Cruciate Ligament (ACL) Injury

Anterior cruciate ligament injury (injury to the ligament on the front of the inside of the knee) is primarily a result of a sudden twisting or hyperextension of the knee. Approximately 70 percent of all traumatic knee injuries are of the anterior cruciate ligament. They occur most frequently during sports that require the foot to be planted while the body changes direction rapidly. For instance, if a skier falls, while her body cuts sharply to the right or left, the skis may keep her feet planted either forward or in the opposite direction from her body, forcing the knee joint into extreme torsion (twisting) and stretching or tearing the ACL. In basketball, the problem of extreme torsion is often exacerbated by hyperextension of the knee while landing from a jump. Injuries range from straining or bruising to a partial, or at worst complete, tearing of the ligament.

Another, less common, cause of ACL injuries is a direct blow, for example, if the knee is slammed into the dashboard during a car accident or is hit in a high-contact sport such as football.

One of the most brutal knee injuries is O'Donoghue's triad. Occurring most often on the football field, this injury results when a player is hit from the side, leading to a series of tears: an ACL rupture plus tears of the medial meniscus and the medial collateral ligament.

The severity of ligament injuries is graded on a scale of one to four:

1. First-degree sprain is an acute mild trauma. A few ligamentous fibers have been torn, resulting in mild pain but no joint instability.
2. Second-degree sprain is an acute moderate trauma. A moderate number of ligamentous fibers are torn, resulting in moderate pain, swelling, and disability but little or no joint instability.
3. Third-degree sprain is an acute and complete tear of the ligament. Swelling and pain may range from minimal to severe. Disability is always severe, and the joint is rendered unstable.
4. Fourth-degree sprain is a complete rupture between the ligament and the bone. Pain, swelling, and disability are severe, and the joint is rendered unstable.

The immediate symptoms indicating that you have suffered an ACL injury vary according to the degree of injury involved. The most common immediate symptom is a loud pop that you both feel and hear. Next your knee may give way.

Frequently you are rendered immobile by an ACL injury. Even if you can move a little, you certainly cannot continue the activity that caused the injury. Your knee may begin to swell immediately and continue to do so until reaching its worst state 2 to 3 hours after the damage was first done. Even if the injury is mild enough to allow you to stand, your knee may feel unstable as if it wants to bend too far back.

The first thing to do if you believe you have suffered an ACL injury is to stop all activity. For some immediate relief employ the treatment commonly referred to as *RICE*: *r*est, *i*ce, *c*ompression (Ace bandage), and elevation (see chapter 5). The next step is a trip to the emergency room, where your knee may be X-rayed and immobilized in a brace.

Medial Collateral Ligament (MCL) Injury

Medial collateral ligament injury (injury to the ligament on the inner side of the knee outside the knee joint) primarily results from an outside blow, such as a tackle from the side in football. This ligament is more easily injured than the ACL, but the injury is far less common than an ACL rupture because most of us don't engage in activities that would put us on the receiving end of such a blow. MCL injury may be caused by a valgus stress, which means the knee is pushed inward (knock-knees are a valgus deformity).

The immediate symptoms that you have incurred an MCL injury may be a pop that you both feel and hear, frequently followed by the knee buckling inward, followed by swelling within several hours. While painful, an MCL injury may not be as serious as an ACL injury, because the other important knee stabilizers often remain intact.

If you believe you have an MCL injury, take the precautions outlined in the previous section for an ACL rupture: RICE and a visit to the emergency room.

Lateral Collateral Ligament (LCL) Injury

Lateral collateral ligament injury (injury to the ligament on the outer side of the knee outside the knee joint) occurs from a varus stress applied from the inside that forces the knee toward the outside. The immediate symptoms and treatment are the same as for MCL injuries.

Posterior Cruciate Ligament (PCL) Injury

Posterior cruciate ligament injuries (injury to the ligament inside the joint and behind the ACL) also occur far less often than ACL injuries. They may result from a direct blow to the bent knee, for example, in a car accident, if your knee hits the dashboard just below the patella (kneecap), or if you fall onto your bent knee. This impact forces the tibia backward on the femur, tearing the PCL. An impact of the sort necessary to create a PCL injury frequently results in the injury of other ligaments as well.

Pain, swelling, buckling of the knee, and a sense of knee instability are symptomatic when you suffer a PCL injury. If you are not properly treated, pain and swelling may be gone in two to four weeks, but knee instability may remain.

If you believe you have suffered a PCL injury, you should immediately follow the RICE protocol (see chapter 5) and visit the doctor or emergency room for further treatment.

Meniscal Injury

Meniscal injuries damage the cushioning tissue between the tibia and the femur, inside the knee joint, on both sides (medial and lateral) of the knee. The menisci are two crescent-shaped discs that act as shock absorbers and enhance knee stability. They are highly vulnerable to injury from abrupt rotations of the knee while it is bearing weight, for example, when you turn to hit a tennis ball, rotating your thigh (femur) while leaving your foot stationary.

If your injury is slight (a small tear or bruise), the menisci will continue to work as a single unit to provide a proper cushion and a sliding surface for the femur and the tibia. However, if you incur a large meniscal tear, a piece of a meniscus can break loose and act as a foreign body inside the joint, causing the knee to catch and lock (when large, this is called a *bucket-handle tear*). This can be extremely painful and debilitating. (See Figure 2.1.)

With a minor injury of the menisci you may experience some pain when you move the knee, but usually you can continue with your activity. If ignored, the initial pain may abate but erupt again later and lead to more severe degeneration. With a severe injury of the meniscus—for example, if a meniscal fragment catches between the femur and the tibia—you will have extreme pain and may have swelling or bleeding in the knee. Over time, you may develop arthritis in the affected area. Unfortunately, removal of the meniscal fragment may also increase your chances of arthritis by leaving less cushion between the bones.

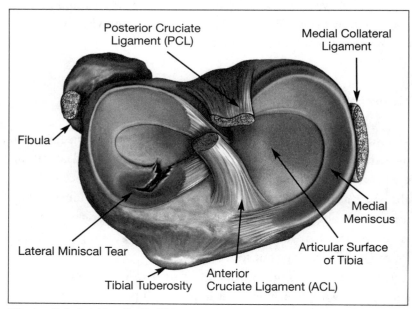

Figure 2.1: Looking Down Through the Injured Knee

Years ago, the entire meniscus was often removed after an injury. Individuals who underwent this procedure usually became severely arthritic and debilitated, and many required knee replacement surgery.

If you believe you have suffered a minor injury to the menisci, follow the RICE regimen (see chapter 5), and visit a physical medicine and rehabilitation specialist (physiatrist) or orthopedic surgeon.

Dislocation of the Patella

Patellar dislocation (displacement of the kneecap from its normal position) may occur from either (1) an abrupt change of direction during high-impact activity such as running, or (2) a direct blow to the patella, such as might occur in an accident. Occasionally, this dislocation occurs from a slight pressure on the patella either during sex or when a dog or child jumps or leans on the knee.

If you dislocate your patella, you will have immediate pain and be unable to move your knee. The kneecap may be visibly off to the side. Swelling and tenderness may occur as the kneecap shifts laterally. It is a very shocking injury.

If you believe you have dislocated your patella, follow the RICE protocol (see chapter 5) and then go immediately to the doctor for treatment. Although I don't recommend it, some people punch their patella back into place.

Rupture of the Patellar Tendon

A ruptured patellar tendon may occur from either an abrupt trauma or long-term tendinitis (inflammation of the tendon), which can weaken the tendon and make it vulnerable to tearing.

Inflammation of the patellar tendon is called *jumper's knee*, because the muscle contraction and force of hitting the ground in jump-heavy sports such as basketball put particular strain on this tendon.

If you rupture your patellar tendon you will not only suffer considerable pain but also have difficulty walking. You may feel a gap above or below the patella. An immediate visit to your doctor is recommended.

Fracture

A fracture (a break in the bone) is usually caused by trauma such as an accident or fall. Occasionally, cancer that either originates in or spreads from elsewhere to the bone may cause a fracture. The immediate signs (visible evidence) and symptoms (evidence that is felt) include pain, inability to move the knee, bones out of anatomical alignment, swelling, bruising, and tenderness. A compound fracture is one in which the bone sticks through the skin.

If you believe you have a fracture, stop moving and seek immediate medical treatment.

In rare cases, a fracture may create a fat embolus (a plug of fat in a blood vessel) or deep venous thrombus (a clot of blood in a vein). These may cause damage if they travel to the lung to produce a pulmonary embolism (obstruction), a condition that could lead to death.

When dealing with a traumatic knee injury, always keep in mind that more than one structure may be damaged.

Stress Fracture

A stress fracture is a bone disruption that occurs without breaking the outer lining of the bone. It results from the bone's inability to resist the repetitive load it bears from activities such as running, marching, bowling, weight lifting, gymnastics, basketball, football, dancing, and rowing. If you have increased pain with activity and swelling, you might have a stress fracture.

If you think that you may have suffered a stress fracture, consult a doctor immediately. A long period of rest and healing will be required if the diagnosis is positive.

REPETITIVE INJURIES

Patellofemoral Syndrome (Runner's Knee)

Runner's knee is known clinically as patellofemoral syndrome. (Iliotibial band syndrome, described later in this chapter, is also called *runner's knee.*) In this injury, the tendon and the retinaculum (a fibrous band covering the front of the knee), which help keep the kneecap in place, may be too tight when the knee is flexed and may jam the patella into the femoral groove. Or the tendon and retinaculum may stretch out and become inflamed in reaction to the stress of repetitive movement—running, squatting, jumping, or twisting activities. When this happens, tracking of the patella may go slightly off course and drift, slip, or tilt, causing further inflammation. Over time, this patellar condition may begin to erode the cartilage on the undersurface of the kneecap, causing even more abrasion, inflammation, and pain.

One symptom indicating that you may have runner's knee is knee pain that is aggravated by any repetitive movement, particularly stair climbing. The condition is exacerbated by prolonged periods of sitting with the knee flexed, for example, in an airplane or a movie theater (your doctor might call this symptom the *positive theater sign,* meaning that discomfort during long sitting periods is a positive in-dicator of runner's knee). You may also feel the knee catching or slipping.

At the earliest sign of these symptoms, consider resting the knee for a day between runs or other aggravating activities. Icing the knee for 20 minutes after exercise can also be helpful (see chapter 5). A simple strap under the kneecap may alleviate the problem (see chapter 7).

If runner's knee is recurrent, a short course of a nonsteroidal anti-inflammatory drug (NSAID), such as ibuprofen, may be helpful (see chapter 5).

Tendinitis

Tendinitis (inflammation of a tendon) may result from overuse of the tendon during any activity, such as dancing, cycling, or running. Since tendons connect muscles to bones, repetitive contraction of a muscle results in repetitive tension on the tendon and its connection to the bone. With heavy sports activity or repeated motion of any kind, tendons may become inflamed. As we age, our tendons often start to deteriorate, lose some elasticity and hydration, and become more susceptible to injury.

A symptom that you have patellar tendinitis is tenderness at the point where the patellar tendon attaches to the tibia or anywhere on or around the patella. You may also experience pain during fast movement, such as running, walking quickly, or jumping.

If you believe you have tendinitis, apply the RICE protocol, and, if that isn't sufficient, try a short course of NSAIDs (see chapter 5). If your symptoms still do not abate, see a physician to ensure total heal-ing and prevent rupture of the tendons.

Bursitis (Housemaid's Knee)

Bursitis is the result of an injured or overused joint. Points of contact between bones, tendonss, and ligaments are often cushioned by small, fluid-filled sacs called *bursae*. When a joint is overused or injured, the bursae may swell with excess fluid. This creates pressure on the surrounding tissue, causing pain, inflammation, and tenderness. Untreated, this condition may lead to inflammation in the soft tissue, restricting and causing pain with knee motion.

The name *housemaid's knee* was applied because the constant bending and kneeling associated with housecleaning is typical of the activity that causes bursitis. Symptoms include pain and stiffness when bending the knee or kneeling and pain and swelling around, on top of, or just below the knee.

If you believe you have bursitis, immediately cease the activity that prompted the symptoms. Note whether your pain and restriction of movement stop and how long it takes for the symptoms to abate. The RICE protocol (see chapter 5) may be effective. If pain persists, try Tylenol or a brief course of NSAIDs (also discussed in chapter 5). If prolonged kneeling is the culprit, knee pads may be curative.

Iliotibial Band Syndrome

Iliotibial band syndrome (which is also called *runner's knee*) is an inflammatory condition resulting from overuse. The iliotibial band is a strip of fascia, or fibrous tissue, that extends from the side of the pelvis to the outside of the knee. Repeated rubbing of this band over the prominent bone on the outer side of the knee occurs during running (particularly downhill), cycling, stair climbing, and other repetitive activities that continuously flex and extend the knee.

A primary symptom of iliotibial band syndrome is an aching or burning sensation at the side of your knee during activity. Pain may be focused at the side of the knee or may travel up the side of the thigh. When you bend and then straighten the knee, you may feel a snapping sensation. Swelling and difficulty moving the knee are not generally associated with this condition, and these symptoms suggest a different injury.

If you believe you have iliotibial band syndrome, rest the knee to allow time for healing and reduction of the inflammation. Mild stretching may be helpful. To do one simple stretch, lie on the floor and pull the affected leg across your body. You may also try icing after exercise and a short course of NSAIDs, such as ibuprofen (see chapter 5).

Osgood-Schlatter Disease

Osgood-Schlatter disease most commonly affects young people—particularly boys—between the ages of ten and fifteen who play games that include frequent running and jumping, such as basketball. It is caused by repetitive stress or tension on a portion of the growth area of the upper tibia (the tibial tuberosity) just below the knee. The condition is characterized by inflammation of the patellar tendons and surrounding soft tissue where the tendon attaches to the tibia. The pain below the knee joint gets worse with activity and improves with rest. A bony bump that is painful when pressed may appear just below the kneecap. Motion of the knee is not generally affected, but the pain may last for months and recur until the child finishes growing. After healing has occurred, the bony growth remains, although it is not painful.

If you suspect you have Osgood-Schlatter disease, rest and ice your knee. Standard treatments are discussed in chapter 6 and rehabilitation protocols in chapter 7. In addition to reduced activity, nutritional therapy with selenium and vitamin E and prolotherapy injections are helpful (see chapter 8).

Chapter Three

Pathological Conditions and Syndromes

Some repetitive injuries to the knee worsen into conditions known as overuse or repetitive stress syndromes. One example is plica syndrome. Other conditions of the knee are of pathological origin, although repetitive stress contributes to them. These include osteochondritis dissecans, several types of arthritis, chondromalacia patellae, and gout.

PLICA SYNDROME

Plica syndrome consists of irritation and inflammation of the plica. The plica is a band of remnant synovial tissue (a thin, slippery material that lines all of the joints) that is left over from the earliest stages of fetal development. Generally, as a fetus matures, these tissue pouch remnants come together to form one large cavity—the synovial cavity—within the knee. However, in some people the plica does not fuse completely, leaving four folds or bands of plica within the knee instead of one combined cavity.

Overuse and injury may inflame the plica. If you suffer from plica syndrome, you will experience pain, swelling, a clicking sensation, locking, and weakness in your knee.

If you believe you have plica syndrome, reduce your activity, apply ice and compression (an elastic bandage) to your knee, and, if necessary, try a short course of NSAIDs (see chapter 5). Only a doctor can properly and thoroughly diagnose plica syndrome, because its symptoms mimic those of many other knee problems.

OSTEOCHONDRITIS DISSECANS

Osteochondritis dissecans, like Osgood-Schlatter disease (described in chapter 2), is most commonly found in active adolescents or young adults. It results from a loss of blood supply to the area of bone beneath a joint surface; this may be due to a slight blockage of a small artery, an unrecognized injury, or a minuscule fracture that damages the cartilage overlying the joint. The result is avascular necrosis (bone degeneration due to lack of blood supply). Although osteochondritis dissecans most often affects the inner side of the knee at the end of the femur, it may be found in other parts of the knee or other joints as well. As time goes on, the lack of blood causes the affected bone and its cartilage covering to loosen, resulting in pain and possibly severe osteoarthritis.

Locking of the knee joint, weakness, and sharp pain are all symptoms of osteochondritis dissecans. At the onset of such symptoms, visit your doctor for a thorough diagnosis and monitoring. This condition may heal spontaneously. If it doesn't, surgical intervention may be required to inhibit problems later in life. In many cases, stopping repetitive activities is the only positive treatment.

ARTHRITIS

Arthritis is a generic term for inflammation in the joints (*arth* means "joint" and *itis* means "inflammation"). It arises from different etiologies (causes of pathology or disease). Despite the roots of the generic term, the etiologies of certain forms of arthritis are not actually inflammatory but instead traumatic or repetitive in nature.

Osteoarthritis

Osteoarthritis (also called *degenerative arthritis* or *degenerative joint disease*) is the most common form of arthritis. It can occur as ligaments stretch and loosen and as joints become unstable. Bones then move more freely, creating greater friction, which wears away the smooth cartilage protecting the bone. When one bone rubs painfully against another, the joint attempts to stabilize itself by growing more bone and becoming bulkier (a condition known as *hypertrophy*). See Figure 3.1. Another complication common to osteoarthritis of the knee is that small pieces of cartilage break off and float around the knee, causing inflammation, pain, and occasional locking of the joint.

Common signs and symptoms of osteoarthritis include joint pain that increases with activity, weather changes, and rain; stiffness in the joints; loss of movement and dexterity; some swelling and hypertrophy; and often crepitus, a cracking or crunching sound when the joint is moved.

Factors that may contribute to the development of osteoarthritis include obesity, heavy exercise, hard physical labor, trauma, and vitamin D deficiency. Before age forty-five, osteoarthritis is found more commonly in men; after age fifty-five, females are more likely to

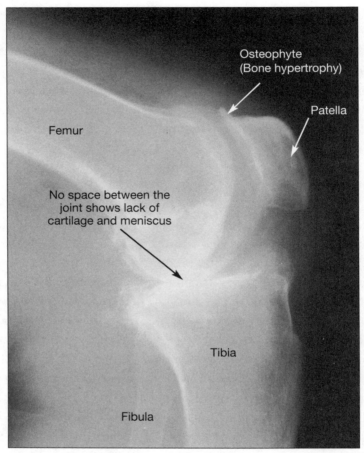

Figure 3.1: Lateral X-Ray View of the Knee Showing Severe Osteoarthritis (Bone on Bone)

develop it. As much as 30 percent of the population may have a genetic predisposition to osteoarthritis.

If you think you have symptoms of osteoarthritis, first reduce your activity and determine whether your symptoms quickly resolve. (Figure 3.2 shows the result of severe, bone on bone, osteoarthritis.) If so,

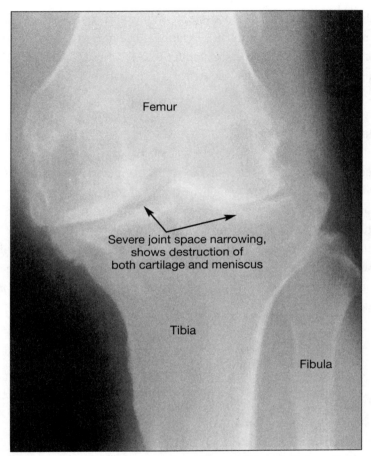

Femur

Severe joint space narrowing,
shows destruction of
both cartilage and meniscus

Tibia

Fibula

Figure 3.2: Frontal X-Ray of the Knee Showing Severe Osteoarthritis
(Bone on Bone)

you may adjust your level of activity to one that keeps your pain tolerable. Many people who suffer from osteoarthritis can modify their activity to live comfortably without medication or medical intervention. Try both ice and heat therapies to see which works best for you. If the pain lingers for days after activity has ceased, try taking natural supplements such as glucosamine sulfate and chondroitin sulfate to inhibit pain (see chapter 8). Tylenol is the next step, and then a short course of (NSAIDs) (see chapter 5). An X ray, CT scan, or MRI can definitively diagnose osteoarthritis (see chapter 4).

Rheumatoid Arthritis

Rheumatoid arthritis is believed to result from an autoimmune dysfunction (a condition in which the body's immune system reacts to its own tissue or cell types as if they were foreign matter) or an infection (viral or bacterial), but its exact etiology has not yet been determined. Whereas osteoarthritis begins in the joint, rheumatoid arthritis originates in the synovial membrane that coats the inside of the joint. It shares many of the symptoms of osteoarthritis, but has these differences:

- With osteoarthritis, pain generally diminishes when activity does, but with rheumatoid arthritis it continues even when the afflicted area is at rest.
- Rheumatoid arthritis may cause a thickening around the joints and is accompanied by general fatigue.
- While osteoarthritis is found only in individual joints and does not spread, rheumatoid arthritis is a systemic condition that may affect many organ systems.

Early warning signs of rheumatoid arthritis include:

- Stiffness in the morning that lasts for more than an hour after rising.
- Fatigue and weight loss.

- Fever, joint pain, and swelling that continue for more than a six-week period.

About 20 percent of rheumatoid arthritis sufferers develop small nodules or lumps beneath the skin.

Consult a doctor if you experience these symptoms, because rheumatoid arthritis is a progressive disease that may be inhibited or stopped by certain drugs: disease-modifying antirheumatic drugs (DMARDs). A blood test for rheumatoid factor may help diagnose the disease.

Immediate relief from symptoms of rheumatoid arthritis may be provided by stopping the activity that began the pain or by immobilizing the joint with an elastic bandage or brace. Whether heat or ice offers relief depends on the stage of the disease. Try both to discover which one works for you. In mild cases, aspirin effectively reduces pain and swelling.

Infectious (Septic) Arthritis

Infectious arthritis (or septic arthritis) results when bacteria invade a joint. This invasion may be direct, such as through a wound, or spread from another part of the body, or spread through blood vessels. As bacteria grow, pus forms in the joint, and redness and swelling develop. Left untreated, infectious arthritis can cause permanent cartilage damage and fusion of the joint.

Signs and symptoms of infectious arthritis include pain, redness, swelling, heat, and tenderness at the knee; fever; and chills. The onset of symptoms may be quite sudden.

If you suffer these symptoms, immediately visit the doctor or emergency room. Septic arthritis is a medical emergency, and delay could have severe consequences: your joint might be destroyed and rendered useless.

CHONDROMALACIA PATELLAE

Chondromalacia patellae is degeneration of the articular cartilage (cartilage that covers bone) on the back of the patella (kneecap). Because the cartilage is impaired, the femur rubs against the patella, rather than gliding smoothly across it, which roughens the patellar cartilage even more.

This condition can be accurately diagnosed using an MRI scan. An X ray is not definitive. It is frequently either overdiagnosed or misdiagnosed as patellofemoral syndrome (runner's knee), a more common condition that may occur *without* cartilage damage.

From 75 to 85 percent of chondromalacia patellae cases are cured by using conservative care for two to six months. Surgery is often not successful.

GOUT

Gout is a joint inflammation resulting from an excess of uric acid in the body. Uric acid is a normal by-product of digestion that is regularly eliminated through urination. A sudden change in uric acid production may lead to an excess of uric acid that the body is unable to eliminate. This excess may crystalize and lodge in the joints, resulting in pain and swelling. Attacks of gout usually recur and, after the second attack, may recur more frequently and last for longer periods of time. Gout signs and symptoms include swollen joints that are tender, hot, and red. The skin over the joint may become shiny and dry, and even the weight of a bedsheet on the joint can be excruciating. Successive gout attacks may destroy a joint.

Gout may be prompted by excessive consumption of alcohol and protein (particularly organ meats, sardines, and anchovies), use of diuretics, obesity, trauma, or surgery.

The pain associated with gout is so severe that you will need no prompting to visit a doctor immediately.

This chapter has discussed many types of knee pathologies and conditions. The next chapter takes you through the steps required to make a firm diagnosis and determine a course of treatment.

Chapter Four

Examination and Diagnosis of the Painful Knee

Once you have taken the initial steps to keep from making a bad knee problem worse, put yourself in the hands of experts. Since nothing is more frightening than the unknown, this chapter is designed to send you into the doctor's office as prepared as possible. You'll learn about the questions, physical examinations, and medical procedures commonly used in making a complete and accurate diagnosis of knee problems.

THE HISTORY OF YOUR KNEE

The first thing the doctor will want you to do is answer a number of questions about your knee. It's important to give answers that are as complete as possible. Just because you're in the office as a result of a skiing accident, don't assume that previous injuries or symptoms are unimportant. Standard inquiries about the state of your knee include the following:

1. What are you able to do, not able to do, and able to do only with difficulty? Consider the following actions: bending or straightening your knee, running, walking, jumping, hill climbing and descending, stair climbing and descending, sitting or standing for prolonged periods, getting to your feet after long periods of sitting.

2. Are you experiencing pain? Where precisely is it located? Is it a sharp pain or a dull ache? Is it constant or intermittent? Is it associated with a particular activity or activities? Does it begin after activity has ceased? If so, about how long after that cessation?

3. Is your pain or discomfort worse in the morning or at night? Consider possible adjustments that could be made in either your sleeping arrangements or your workstation.

4. Do you hear a clicking or grating sound around the affected area? If you had a traumatic injury, did you hear a pop at the time it occurred?

5. Does your knee give way or catch? If so, is there a particular activity (such as stepping from a curb) that instigates it?

6. Has your gait (manner of walking) been affected by your knee problem? Have you had any gait-related problems or injuries in your past?

7. Have you ever injured your knee before? (Even if the injury wasn't recent, it might be relevant. Don't dismiss an incident just because you don't think it's important.) Even without injury, have you previously experienced even minor knee pain or weakness?

8. If you suffered a trauma, how did the accident or incident occur? Did you receive a blow of some kind? Was the knee bearing weight at the time of injury—for instance, were you running (weight-bearing) as opposed to driving a car (not weight-bearing)?

9. Did your knee become swollen, red, or warm as a result of your injury? Have you had similar signs in the knee on any previous occasion? Have you had a fever?

10. What type of footwear did you have on at the time of the incident? What type of shoes do you usually wear? Do you use any sort of orthotics (shoe inserts), either prescribed

or over-the-counter (such as Dr. Scholl's)? Be sure to bring your shoes and orthotics with you to your doctor.

11. What is your regular exercise regime? Does it require special shoes? If so, how regularly do you replace or refurbish them?

12. What actions (if any) have you taken regarding your knee from the time you either suffered injury or began to be bothered by your knee until your arrival in the emergency room or doctor's office?

OBSERVING KNEE FUNCTION

Once the doctor has taken a history, she will start the examination by taking a good look at the problem. You need to remove any clothing that interferes with viewing or examining your knee. If possible, the doctor will stand so that she may observe whether your posture is straight-legged, bowlegged, or knock-kneed and whether the knee can bear weight. The doctor will also check for any visible anomalies, such as swelling, discoloration, bony protrusions, or small lumps around or behind your knee.

Next, the doctor will observe you on the examination table. If only one knee is injured, the doctor will examine the "normal" one first to determine your usual knee function for comparison. Then your injured knee will be bent at a 90-degree angle, with your foot flat on the table, so that the examiner can observe whether the knee is properly aligned in a relaxed bent position.

MOVING THE KNEE

The examiner will next check the knee for movement. This is done in two ways. First, you may be asked to move the knee. From a sitting position on the examining table, you will extend your leg, or lying on your back on the table with your knee bent you will rotate it outward and inward or bend and straighten your leg or make other movements. Second, you will remain passive while the examiner manipulates your knee through an extensive series of movements.

If you are able to move and have your knee manipulated with relative ease and minimal discomfort, you may be asked to perform functional movement tests such as running, jumping, or walking.

Much of knee diagnosis is truly "hands on." The skilled examiner tests for muscle resistance, checks for ligament laxity, searches for lumps or swelling, rotates joints to assess flexibility, determines your strength and range of movement—all with the touch of his hands.

Sometimes in the course of the examination the doctor is required to extend or manipulate your knee in a way that temporarily causes pain. The Drawer test or Lachman's test is used to assess anterior cruciate ligament (ACL) competence by attempting to sublux the femur from the tibia. Nobody enjoys being hurt, but try to exhale with the pain and go with it, because finding that "pain point" is often key to a successful diagnosis and is a necessary evil on the road to getting you well.

DETERMINING THE NEXT STEP

Several things may happen after the initial examination.

- A diagnosis may be reached and subsequent course of action decided upon.
- A preliminary diagnosis may be made, along with a decision to "wait and see" how the knee progresses. Rest and some support from a brace, crutches, or the like may be prescribed.

• Additional medical diagnostic procedures may be initiated immediately. These may be simple office procedures or advanced techniques using the latest marvels in diagnostic equipment. Various options are described next.

KNEE ASPIRATION

Draining the knee (knee aspiration) may be indicated when swelling is present. An immediate, tense swelling that occurs within 2 hours of knee injury usually indicates that there is blood in the joint (a hemarthrosis, often the result of a torn ACL). If swelling occurs hours later or the next day, it generally indicates fluid resulting from a slower bleed (often a meniscal tear). If you have a systemic bleeding disorder, knee swelling may result from bleeding after even a mild trauma.

Inserting a needle and draining the fluid is useful for both you and your doctor. It provides you with immediate relief from swelling and pain; and it helps the doctor confirm the diagnosis by the presence or absence of blood, pus, or gout crystals in the fluid.

Draining the knee may be useful in diagnosing the following problems:

• Cruciate ligament injuries
• Meniscal injuries
• Bursitis
• Infection
• Osteoarthritis
• Hemophilia
• Sickle-cell anemia
• Fracture
• Gout

If blood is present in the drained fluid, about 70 percent of the time the injury involves a torn ACL. Blood may also indicate a fracture. If bacteria can be cultured from the joint fluid, an infection is present. If the fluid is clear and straw-colored, it may indicate osteoarthritis. A certain kind of crystal found in the fluid indicates gout.

X RAYS

An X ray shows bone photographically and may be used to confirm (or eliminate) a fracture diagnosis. X rays may also reveal chipping in the bone joint surface. Because the ligaments, tendons, joint capsule, and muscles (soft tissue) are not visible in an X ray, its usefulness in diagnosing knee injuries is limited.

An X ray may be useful in diagnosing the following:

- Fractures
- Patellofemoral syndrome
- Arthritis
- Osteochondritis dissecans
- Bone disease
- Osteoporosis

COMPUTERIZED TOMOGRAPHY (CT) SCANS

A computerized tomography scan is a procedure that combines a number of X-ray pictures with computer enhancement to generate cross-sectional views (and, if necessary, three-dimensional images) of the internal structures and organs of the body. Dye may be injected into the damaged structure to illuminate the pathology and enhance the picture. The dye may indicate a tumor or determine bone or soft-tissue involvement in the injury.

CT scans are useful in clearly defining complicated fractures or viewing structures deep within the body. To picture the type of image recorded by a CT scan, imagine your body as a loaf of sliced bread. The scanned photos enable you to see the surface of each slice, even though the loaf remains whole.

Although CT scans use a considerably higher level of radiation than traditional X rays, they pose no discernible risk. However, some patients have reactions to the dye injection—at minimum a feeling of warmth and slight itching, at maximum an extreme allergic reaction, which may inhibit breathing. The latter is generally a result of iodine allergy (iodine is the basis of some dyes). If you are concerned about allergy, be certain to tell your doctor before the procedure.

CT scanning requires that you lie still on a mobile table, which is then moved at small intervals through the scanner, an open-ended tube that looks sort of like an extended doughnut.

Each image takes a few seconds to record, and the entire scan takes several minutes. If you are agitated by the need to remain so still, you may be given a sedative.

A CT scan is useful in diagnosing bone pathology in greater detail than an X ray or MRI.

MAGNETIC RESONANCE IMAGING (MRI)

Magnetic resonance imaging is used not only in diagnostic orthopedics but also in other fields of medicine. An MRI allows doctors to take a picture of the cross section of any part of the body and observe some tissues in far greater detail than is possible with an X ray or CT scan. (See Figure 4.1.)

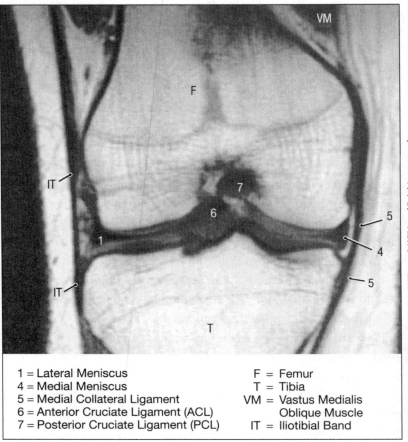

1 = Lateral Meniscus   F = Femur
4 = Medial Meniscus   T = Tibia
5 = Medial Collateral Ligament   VM = Vastus Medialis
6 = Anterior Cruciate Ligament (ACL)   Oblique Muscle
7 = Posterior Cruciate Ligament (PCL)   IT = Iliotibial Band

Figure 4.1: MRI Showing Frontal View of the Knee

Unlike a CT scanner or X-ray machine, an MRI machine does not expose you to radiation. In simplest terms, the machine uses a magnetic field to pass a force through molecules. This passage creates an "excited" stage in the molecules. When the molecules finish reacting to that stage and return to rest, a very detailed image of the area results.

To undergo the MRI, you lie on a flat, mobile bed that is then slid into a body-length tubelike cylinder. A potential problem is that the cylinder can feel extremely claustrophobic. Patient reactions range from mild discomfort to panic attack. It's important to inform your physician if you have a history of claustrophobia or panic attacks. You may be given a sedative before the scan is performed. A newer model of MRI equipment is not a complete tube and thus offers more open area around the patient. This machine is frequently used for claustrophobic patients or patients weighing more than 275 pounds, who are generally not able to fit into the traditional MRI model. The drawback to the more open model is that the picture it generates may not be as clear, because the recording coil that creates the picture operates more effectively the closer it is to the body.

An MRI is particularly useful in knee diagnosis because it offers detailed pictures of ligaments, menisci, and tendons as well as bones. Injuries to those soft tissues are not visible through other procedures.

If you have a pacemaker, have metal clips at the base of your brain as a result of aneurysm repair, work with a lathe, or have any type of metal implant, you may not be able to have an MRI. If you have ever had these, or metal debris in your eye, or any metal residue or fragment in your body, be certain to inform your physician. Metal can be pulled loose by the magnetic force.

An MRI is useful in diagnosing almost any knee condition. Unfortunately it is very expensive.

ARTHROSCOPY

Arthroscopy is a technological marvel that allows the doctor to literally see into the knee (*arthro* means "joint" and *scope* means "to see"). When other examinations fail to find the problem, diagnostic arthroscopy is used to find it and cure it at the same time. (See Figure 4.2.)

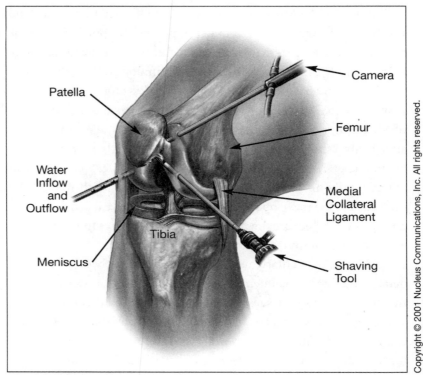

Patella

Camera

Femur

Water
Inflow
and
Outflow

Medial
Collateral
Ligament

Tibia

Meniscus

Shaving
Tool

Figure 4.2: Arthroscopic Surgery

The arthroscope works as follows: Two to four tiny incisions
(ports) are made at strategic points around the knee. Through one
port, instruments are inserted; through another, a small fiber-optic
TV camera. The additional incisions facilitate fluid drainage or the
insertion of additional instruments if called for. Sterile fluid is then
pumped into the knee, enlarging the knee joint so that the camera
and instruments can fit into the space, and keeping the camera lens
clear and free of debris. The instruments are then used to probe, cut,
and smooth various structures, allowing the doctor a full view of the

anatomy and injury as she works. Arthroscopic techniques are not used merely to diagnose injuries but also to repair them.

This chapter described diagnostic techniques that are common in traditional Western medicine. They are procedures you will commonly encounter on a trip to the orthopedic surgeon or emergency room. Prolotherapy, acupuncture, and other alternative forms of diagnosis and treatment are detailed in chapter 8.

Chapter Five

Repairing the Knee

Your injury has been diagnosed, and treatment is being considered. If I could impress one thing upon you at this stage, it would be this: *Go slowly*. Surgery should be a last resort—not a first choice.

PROCEEDING CONSERVATIVELY

In most cases, pursuing rest and rehabilitation first, even if you ultimately decide upon surgery, can only be to your benefit. In fact, even complete ACL ruptures heal faster after surgery if the procedure is postponed.

There are some traumatic injuries for which surgery is often recommended: a complete tear of a ligament or tendon, and a fracture that leaves the joint unstable or out of correct anatomical position. Even so, lag time may occur between diagnosis and surgery, during which your knee is immobilized, and swelling is allowed to diminish. Use that time to make sure you're in the best possible hands. Even though a course of treatment is a given, the person in charge of that course of treatment should, as much as possible, be someone with whom you have great confidence and open, full communication.

Find out what you can about the doctor's surgical history. Also talk about postoperative recovery. You want a surgeon who will tell you honestly about the time and degree of commitment you'll need for successful recuperation and full rehabilitation. If the specialist does not make these facts clear, you may face an unexpected and arduous process; you might want a second opinion. The head of orthopedic surgery at a university is often a good choice. Or ask your surgeon who he would use if his knee were injured.

This chapter explores the standard treatment options offered by orthopedic surgeons and traditional Western medicine, beginning with the least invasive procedures and ending with surgery, the most extreme option. Alternative and newly evolving treatments are outlined in chapter 8.

THE RICE PROTOCOL

The immediate treatment for knee injuries has been given the acronym *RICE*—it consists of *r*est, *i*ce, *c*ompression, and *e*levation In most instances, sprains, strains, and tears are so minor that this regimen will do the trick.

You should rest the knee for as long as it takes to resolve the worst of the condition. Apply ice for no more than 20 minutes in an hour, continuing the applications as needed for the first 72 hours. After that you may apply heat or ice as you prefer. Use constant compression on the knee until the swelling starts to go down. An elastic bandage is the simplest method to use. Wrap it as firmly as you can tolerate without pain. Elevate your knee above the level of your heart, if possible, to help fluid leave the knee and return to your circulatory system.

NONSTEROIDAL
ANTI-INFLAMMATORY DRUGS (NSAIDs)

If your injury is minor, all you may need in addition to the RICE protocol is a short course of nonsteroidal anti-inflammatory drugs, such as aspirin, ibuprofen, Motrin, Daypro, Naprosyn, Celebrex, or Vioxx. (Acetaminophen—Tylenol—is not an anti-inflammatory, just a great pain reliever. Because of the side effects of NSAIDs, try using Tylenol first.) For chronic conditions, such as rheumatoid arthritis, a controlled, ongoing course of NSAIDs or other drugs may be the primary course of treatment.

It is important to stress that, while NSAIDs do reduce inflammation and pain, are commonly available in their over-the-counter form, and are used regularly, they are not risk-free. They inhibit the body's production of prostaglandins, and, while prostaglandins cause inflammation, they also protect the stomach lining from the acid that causes ulcers. Overuse of NSAIDs could cause a bleeding ulcer by inhibiting the gastrointestinal protection that prostaglandins provide. In an extreme circumstance, overuse of NSAIDs could lead to death by bleeding, so check with your doctor about drug protocols, and don't take two different NSAIDs at the same time.

People who are elderly; have a history of peptic ulcers; are regular users of antacids, H2 blockers, or omeprazole; or have a history of stomach problems should consult a doctor before using NSAIDs. People who use tobacco and alcohol regularly are also advised to be careful about NSAID consumption. If you are on any course of prescription drugs, consult your doctor or pharmacist before taking even the mildest over-the-counter medication.

The next step after these preliminary treatments is likely to be immobilization of the knee.

KNEE BRACES AND IMMOBILIZATION

The knee may be immobilized in several ways: by wearing an elastic bandage or full-knee brace (most commonly); or through application of a removable splint or cast.

Elastic Bandages

The least intrusive, and most readily available, brace is an elastic (Ace) bandage. It may be used to inhibit daily movement or a specific activity. By limiting your range of motion, an elastic bandage helps reduce swelling (it inhibits motion-induced inflammation) and promotes healing (it protects the sprained or strained ligaments or tendons from further actions and impacts that could extend or increase the damage). An elastic bandage is also used to compress the knee and stop further fluid accumulation.

Full-Knee Braces

Braces are used for two purposes: (1) to protect your knee while healing after injury, and (2) to keep an injury or repetitive condition from becoming worse. The type of brace depends on its purpose.

A protective knee brace, such as an ACL brace, is generally worn when the knee is in motion and is often used in conjunction with crutches. Properly used, it gives the knee the optimum chance to heal from tears, strains, and sprains. Whether you undergo rehabilitation and recovery, as opposed to surgery, often depends on your willingness to listen to and follow your doctor's directions for using a knee brace. The more complex braces must be fitted by a certified orthotist, a physical therapist, or a physician. They are not available over the counter in drugstores or medical supply stores.

Another form of knee brace is used for repetitive injury conditions such as patellofemoral syndrome (runner's knee). The brace keeps your patella in place with external support from either a Velcro band below the patella or a sleeve with a hole that the patella fits into. Without these, the patella may slip and shift, creating abrasion and inflammation. External braces can control that slippage, allowing you to function normally and inhibiting the damage that irregular patellar movement may cause.

Casts

A cast is used for a fracture or other problem in which the joint must be completely immobilized. Modern casts are made of moldable fiberglass and are worn until the problem subsides. For fractures, usually six to eight weeks are required.

If your knee cannot move through its full range of motion (ROM), your doctor may apply serial casting. The bent knee is placed in a cast for a week or so; then the cast is removed, the knee is bent farther, and another cast is applied. This is repeated until you attain the desired ROM.

Casts have several disadvantages: They are bulky. You may need to use crutches for ambulation with a cast, and crutches can be uncomfortable and difficult to use, causing pain in the arms, neck, and back. Total immobilization in a cast for weeks causes profound muscle atrophy. It is difficult to scratch the itchy skin underneath a cast (some people use hangers or knitting needles). It is difficult to watch for possible infection underneath a cast. And casts can cause constriction if applied too tightly.

CORTISONE (CORTICOSTEROID)

If RICE, NSAIDs, and immobilization fail to diminish your knee pain and inflammation sufficiently, a direct injection of cortisone (corticosteroid) into the injured area may be necessary.

Cortisone is a powerful anti-inflammatory available under such prescription names as Depo-Medrol and Celestone. Anti-inflammatory steroids may be taken orally or through skin application, but injection is the most common route of application when treating the knee. In some cases an injection may provide months or years of relief for osteoarthritis. For conditions such as bursitis and tendinitis, in which tissue inflammation is localized to a small area, a steroid injection may resolve the problem. Don't confuse this type of steroid with the kind ingested in large doses by weight lifters. It won't build any muscle for you.

In general, steroid injections treat specific areas of inflammation, such as the part of the knee with bursitis, tendinitis, or arthritis. Occasionally steroids are taken orally to treat systemic conditions such as rheumatoid arthritis.

Steroid injections are easily administered in a doctor's office. Benefits manifest rapidly with only a single injection, and you may avoid the potential side effects of other anti-inflammatories or oral steroids, such as stomach irritation. Oral steroids may produce myriad serious side effects, including psychosis, hypertension, and avascular necrosis of the hip.

Steroid injections do have their own potential for side effects, however. Lesser problems include soreness, discoloration or dimpling of the skin, and localized bleeding from broken blood vessels at the injection site. More severe complications include possible tendon weakening or rupture from multiple injections in or near the tendon. A rule of thumb is to limit steroid injections in a single area to three per year.

Diabetes patients should exercise caution if receiving a steroid injection, because it may transiently raise blood sugar. It could also exacerbate active infection or, by fighting localized inflammation, mask general signs of inflammation and other symptoms in individuals who are suffering from an infection but have not yet been diagnosed.

SURGICAL OPTIONS

If other treatments fail, your doctor may recommend a knee operation. Surgery is not a guarantee of cure, and postoperative rehabilitation is mandatory. The better shape you're in going into surgery, the better shape you're likely to be in coming out of it. Since postoperative pain and swelling limit motion, your muscles may atrophy quickly. It's best to have muscles strong prior to surgery. To regain full strength and full range of motion quickly, you must be willing to work hard after surgery. If you do so, usually you'll recover well. If you do not follow instructions, you're likely to have a poor outcome. That having been said, let us review the common procedures, pros and cons, and likely outcomes of standard knee surgery.

Arthroscopy

Arthroscopy was discussed in chapter 4 as a diagnostic technique that also serves as a treatment. Briefly, a camera and operating tools are inserted through small incisions into the knee joint. The surgeon can then view the interior of the joint on a TV monitor. This allows him to diagnose—and operate on—the problem areas.

An arthroscopic examination may reveal:

- Inflammation in the lining (synovium) of the knee
- Tears in the menisci
- Wearing down of the articular cartilage
- Tears in the ACL and PCL
- Arthritis
- Loose and floating fragments of bone and cartilage
- Patellofemoral syndrome
- Plica syndrome
- Joint fractures

Arthroscopic surgery as a treatment generally involves either repair or removal. The remarkable advantage of arthroscopy is, of course, that it requires the least possible invasion. When repairing a tear, the tiny instruments used in arthroscopy can stitch up the affected area with minimal trauma to surrounding ligaments, tendons, and other tissues. (Before arthroscopy techniques were used, the surgeon had to make major invasive incisions in the knee, often with mixed results and significant potential for operative harm.)

When tissue is to be removed, surgeons now realize that less is more. Previously, removal of damaged structures was thought to be the best treatment for knee problems. Surgeons now believe that all components of the knee are vital to stability, and that removal of any cushion can promote arthritis and its chronic pain. Removing only small sections of injured areas minimizes the potential for surgically induced harm that might necessitate a knee replacement later. Arthroscopy also allows a surgeon to remove tiny bone and cartilage fragments that may be the cause of irritation and inflammation, while disrupting the surrounding structures as little as possible.

Because incisions and invasion are minimized, recovery time for arthroscopic surgery is much less than for more invasive procedures.

Nonetheless, in arthroscopic surgery, like any surgery, complications are possible, including infection, development of a deep venous thrombus (blood clot), an allergic reaction to the anesthetic, vulnerability to reinjury, or failure to repair the problem. If you experience any postoperative pain, swelling, redness, drainage, bleeding, fever, or other symptoms of infection, notify your physician immediately.

Meniscal Repair

Repair of a meniscus is frequently done by arthroscopy, but traditional surgical procedures with a large incision are still used in some instances. Trauma, twisting, and repetitive motion (such as squatting or kneeling) may result in meniscal tears.

Depending on the extent of the injury, one of two surgical options may be advised: repair or removal. In a repair, the meniscus is stitched together again. This can be effective only if the tear is near the perimeter of the meniscus, which has a blood supply to promote healing. Arthroscopic sewing techniques are continually improving and with them the opportunity for restoring the menisci.

If a meniscus is severely damaged, removal may be called for. Years ago, surgeons usually removed the entire meniscus if a tear was found. They now realize that this wholesale removal causes many long-term problems. Orthopedists are just beginning to understand the role of the menisci in stabilizing the knee. Removal of this protective disc leads to irritation and may promote arthritis, chronic discomfort, and pain. Rather than removing the disc, surgeons now perform what is known as a *partial meniscectomy*, removing only the damaged section of the meniscus, as opposed to the complete disc.

In recent years surgeons have increasingly turned to meniscal transplantation for patients whose menisci have been entirely removed. The transplant comes from a deceased human donor. The primary benefit of the procedure is pain relief. The meniscus is a load-bearing structure capable of supporting 70 percent of the load transmitted through the lateral compartment of the knee and approximately 50 percent medially. It is also believed to provide both nutritional and lubricating benefit to the knee. Its absence creates undue stress on the remaining structures, causing pain. If the ACL is deficient, lack of a meniscus may also result in instability.

If you are a candidate for meniscal transplantation, youth is an advantage, and, what's more important, your knee should be relatively sound physiologically, with articular cartilage intact, no major joint deterioration, and normal knee alignment. Your discomfort should be directly linked to the meniscal removal rather than to other factors. Active patients whose meniscal surgery was relatively recent make ideal candidates. If you qualify, meniscal transplantation can save you a lifetime of potential pain, joint deterioration, and joint replacement.

Generally, you need not be hospitalized for the recovery phase after meniscal repair. Bring any unexpected symptoms or discomfort after surgery to your doctor's attention immediately.

ACL Reconstructive Surgery

Anterior cruciate ligament (ACL) reconstructive surgery is deemed necessary in a variety of circumstances:

- Some surgeons believe that a complete rupture or tear makes the surgery a requirement, not a choice.
- If you have obvious knee instability, and no less than 100 percent return of knee function after injury will do (this is particularly true for young or professional athletes), a rehabilitative course might not be sufficient after traumatic injury, even if the ACL did not suffer a complete tear.

In these cases ACL reconstruction is an important option. A similar injury in an older person with a more sedentary lifestyle or more recreational approach to activity would likely not warrant ACL reconstructive surgery.

- If the ACL remains abnormally lax after some recuperation, creating extreme knee instability, reconstruction may be the appropriate course of action. Keep in mind that many ACL tears do not create an unstable knee, and many people participate in athletic life with a deficient ACL.

Surgeons have long been trying to perfect ACL reconstruction. Early attempts to simply stitch the torn ligament together were usually unsuccessful. The current technique in ACL reconstruction uses a piece of tendon or ligament, either harvested from the patient (a graft) or transplanted from a deceased donor (an allograft). One of the most commonly used tendons for this procedure is a strip of the patellar tendon. Another common graft combines tendons from two of the hamstring muscles that attach to the tibia just below the knee joint—the gracilis and semitendinosis muscles. Studies show that removal of these tendons only minimally affects leg strength, because other larger and stronger muscles can easily assume their function. The surgeon and the patient determine together which type of graft will be used.

The procedure is usually performed by arthroscopy (described earlier in this chapter), in which small incisions are made but the joint itself is not opened. Typically, the surgeon first removes the torn ends of the damaged ligament. If the surgeon will use the patellar tendon, only the middle third of the length of the tendon is used. Two bone plugs (small pieces of bone) are removed, usually one from the tibia and the other from the patella, holes are drilled in the ends of the plugs, and sutures attach the graft to the plugs through these holes. Next, the knee is prepared to accept the graft. Holes are drilled where the ACL formerly inserted into the femur and the tibia. The bone plugs of the graft are inserted into those holes, and the graft is pulled into place and adjusted for the proper tension. Then screws secure the bone plugs in position.

If an allograft is used, it is taken from a tissue bank. The advantage of an allograft is that your own tissue is not removed or disturbed. The allograft operation is shorter because the time required to harvest a graft from your own body is eliminated. Whenever foreign tissue is introduced into the body, there is some chance of rejection. However, because this tissue has been checked for bacteria, stored, and frozen (and is far cleaner than a live transplant), incidence of tissue rejection is rare.

As the graft matures after the operation, the new ACL eventually regains blood supply and cells and becomes a living ligament.

Cartilage Transplantation

Cartilage (or chondral) transplantation may be accomplished in several ways. Commonly used procedures are mosaicplasty and autogenous chondrocyte transplantation.

Degeneration and roughening of the glassy-smooth cartilage surface (also known as the *chondral surface*) generally occurs in a slow and painful process involving the whole surface, and it frequently leads to osteoarthritis. However, an acute trauma can cause wear and tear to only a specific area of cartilage. That isolated cartilage lesion may be treated through chondral transplantation.

Mosaicplasty   The surgical procedure known as *mosaicplasty* does indeed create a sort of mosaic in the knee. Small cylindrical pieces of bone with attached cartilage are placed in the defective area. Packed tightly together, they reconstruct the cartilage surface. The plugs are taken from the inner aspect of the knee receiving treatment and are removed from the section of the knee that bears the least weight. This procedure is relatively new, so follow-up has been short term, but so far no permanent damage seems to occur to the area from which the bone plugs are harvested.

Autogenous Chondrocyte Transplantation Another technique used to fill cartilage lesions resulting from trauma is autogenous chondrocyte transplantation. This involves two surgeries done several weeks apart. In the first, an arthroscope is used to evaluate the cartilage surface and take samples of the chondral (cartilage) cells. The cells are then sent to a lab and cultured. The resultant millions of cells are suspended in fluid for several weeks. Then the knee is opened again, and the cultured cells are placed in the defective area. The new cells are covered with a thin piece of tissue to keep them in place. After surgery, while the cells take hold and fill in the defect, no weight-bearing is allowed; then it is resumed gradually, starting with a toe touch.

The benefit of this procedure over mosaicplasty is that no bone is harvested; the downside is that two surgeries are required.

Only a specially trained physician who is well acquainted with your medical history and current health status can determine whether either of these procedures will help you.

Microfracture

Microfracture is a surgical technique designed to repair damaged articular cartilage without transplantation. Microfracture is arthroscopic surgery in which a small "pick" (awl) is used to make tiny fractures in the bone where it meets the damaged cartilage. These penetrations create an environment in which new cartilage can grow. Unlike mosaicplasty, the microfracture procedure may be effective in cases of general deterioration of the cartilage surface.

A carefully controlled postoperative regimen is vital to the success of this procedure. Follow-up studies over a period of seven years found that, with proper rehabilitation, the great majority of patients felt improvement in their ability to carry out daily activities and a lessening of pain after microfracture was performed.

Arthroplasty

Arthroplasty is the surgical procedure also known as *joint replacement* (*arthro* means "joint," *plasty* means "surgical shaping"). (See Figure 5.1.) This option comes into play when cartilage deterioration and resultant osteoarthritis have become so severe that you are rendered immobile or suffer constant pain. To be a candidate for such surgery you should be otherwise in good health—both emotionally and physically—because the recovery can be quite arduous.

Mechanics of the Procedure To imagine how this procedure works for the knee, you might picture the process of capping a tooth. In knee replacement, a saw removes the damaged cartilage and a small amount of bone. Traditionally, the ends of the bones are then "capped" with metal alloy that is held in place by medical-quality cement or screws. A plastic liner is placed between the bones to create a smooth gliding surface. The underside of the patella is also replaced with a plastic liner, creating the smooth, gliding surface once provided by cartilage. In some cases, surgeons use a porous material that allows the bone to grow into the new bone cap (as opposed to using metal, which has to be attached to the bone). The porous material seems to work better in younger patients with sturdier bone structure; older patients with diminished bone mass enjoy greater success with metal and cement. The cement allows the older patient to ambulate (walk) sooner.

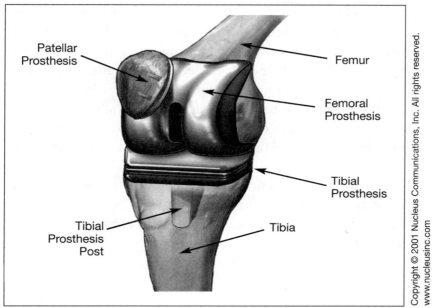

Figure 5.1: Total Knee Replacement

A recent study suggests that some patients may benefit from reconstruction of the medial collateral ligament (MCL) in conjunction with arthroplasty. If a patient has a valgus deformity (knock-knees), is obese, or had previous knee surgeries, the MCL may be so stretched that it offers little support for the new knee. By reconstructing the ligament to offer more support, the surgeon can greatly improve the patient's chance of long-term success.

Risks of Arthroplasty Joint replacement therapy has some grave risks. Like all surgeries, it requires you to weigh the risk factors against the benefits, considering your age, general health, and mobility requirements (active versus sedentary). Proper anticoagulant therapy is essential to reduce the chance of developing a blood clot, which can lead to injury to the lungs or even death. Infection after surgery is rare, but after the metal part is introduced particles may be released that trigger a systemic autoimmune response. In as many as 30 percent of patients, the replacement joint fails after fifteen years; fewer than 10 percent report failure after five years. In a second replacement surgery, patients face a far greater potential for complications than they did in the original procedure—more bone is cut, more blood is lost, and the patient's greater age increases vulnerability to problems.

I admonish younger or very active individuals to wait as long as possible before having a knee replacement. The more activity or trauma a replaced knee undergoes, the sooner a second replacement becomes necessary.

Chapter Six

Standard Treatments for Specific Injuries

Following is a list of the knee conditions outlined in chapters 2 and 3 and the likely course of treatment for each. Medical procedures are described in greater detail in chapter 5. Alternative therapies are discussed in chapter 8.

TRAUMATIC INJURIES

Anterior Cruciate Ligament (ACL) Injury

- Follow the RICE protocol.
- If swelling is severe, the doctor may aspirate your knee (drain fluid from it, using a syringe).
- Wear an ACL brace to stabilize the knee. Used with crutches, it keeps the knee immobilized and allows healing.
- If your symptoms abate and the ligament begins to heal, you may pursue a gentle course of physical therapy to promote healing.
- If your symptoms do not abate (or the original diagnosis was a complete tear of the ACL) and the knee is unstable, ACL reconstructive surgery may be indicated.

Medial Collateral Ligament (MCL) Injury

- Follow the RICE protocol. Apply ice packs to reduce pain and swelling, and wear a small, sleeve-type brace to provide compression and to protect and stabilize the knee.
- If the injury is a sprain rather than a tear in the MCL, combine a prescribed exercise program with an ice pack regimen.
- If the MCL is severely sprained or torn (which may be accompanied by an ACL injury), surgical repair is generally required.

Lateral Collateral Ligament (LCL) Injury

Apply the treatment described in the preceding section for MCL injury but on the lateral (outer) side of the knee.

Posterior Cruciate Ligament (PCL) Injury

- If you suspect a PCL injury, apply the RICE regimen.
- Immobilize the knee with a full leg brace to promote healing.
- If the injury starts to abate, begin a mild course of exercise to restore movement.
- Although PCL injuries are less common than ACL injuries, and more likely to resolve without surgery, surgery is occasionally required. PCL surgical techniques are similar to ACL surgical repairs.

Meniscal Injury

- Follow the RICE protocol, especially rest, and cease strenuous activity.
- If your pain and other symptoms go away, indicating a minor tear, carefully pursue a muscle-strengthening program.
- If your pain and symptoms do not diminish, you may undergo arthroscopy or traditional surgery to repair the injury by suturing (stitching) the meniscus tear.
- If the tear is too extensive to suture, the damaged section may be removed or smoothed surgically.
- As a last resort, if you have suffered a major injury, the surgeon may remove the entire meniscus. This is very rarely done.

Dislocation of the Patella

- Follow the RICE regimen. Apply electrical stimulation to relieve pain and swelling. If the patella pops back into place of its own accord, the RICE protocol is all you need to do.
- If the patella does not go back in place, after the doctor has achieved proper relocation, immobilize the knee in a cylinder cast for three weeks or more.
- If loose and floating fragments have resulted from the injury, you may undergo arthroscopic surgery to remove them, to eliminate pain and inflammation.
- Follow a prescribed rehabilitative course to strengthen the vastus medialis oblique (VMO) muscle and restore its ability to hold the patella in place.

- If the patella goes out of position again after recovery, surgical release of the lateral retinaculum or repositioning of the tendon on the tibia may be indicated.

Rupture of the Patellar Tendon

- Follow the RICE protocol to reduce swelling and prepare for further treatment. A ruptured tendon is extraordinarily painful.
- If you have suffered a partial tear, your knee may be immobilized in a cast.
- If you have suffered a complete tear, your surgeon will reattach the tendon. You then will be put in a cast for six to twelve weeks.
- Follow a prescribed rehabilitation program to increase strength and range of motion.

Fracture

- Go immediately to the doctor or emergency room. On the way, you may begin the RICE protocol. Make no attempt to straighten or adjust the injured knee under any circumstance.
- After confirming the fracture, the surgeon may reset the bones in place using surgical pins or plates. In a fracture with many small breaks, the surgeon may use a bone graft.
- The fractured area may be immobilized in a cast for six to twelve weeks, depending on your recuperative ability and the severity of the injury. Children generally need to spend no more than six weeks in a cast, while older patients with frailer bones may need longer immobilization.

Stress Fracture

- Immediately cease vigorous activity. Often you will not be able to resume activity for weeks.
- Use a cane or crutch to keep weight off the injured knee. Since no muscles or tendons are directly injured in a stress fracture, a cast is not called for unless immobilization is needed to stop activity.
- As your pain lessens and movement becomes easier, begin a series of prescribed exercises to restore the knee completely.

REPETITIVE INJURIES

Patellofemoral Syndrome (Runner's Knee)

Patellofemoral syndrome is a very mild form of patellar dislocation. Nonsurgical interventions include the following:

- Decrease your activity and apply ice to relieve pain and reduce inflammation.
- Apply a simple strap (a Chopat strap, for example, made of Velcro) under the knee or use taping to hold the patella in place in the femoral groove during exercise.
- If the syndrome is chronic, a course of NSAIDs may be prescribed.
- Do exercises to strengthen the vastus medialis oblique muscle (the quadriceps muscle on the inside of the lower thigh), which may pull the patella into its track. Working out on a stationary bike is usually excellent for recovery. It also provides cardiac protection.

In severe cases, surgical intervention—arthroscopic smoothing of the undersurface of the patella—may be required.

Tendinitis

- Follow a regimen of rest, ice, elevation, and immobilization in a removable brace.
- A course of NSAIDs may be prescribed.
- If your inflammation continues, a cortisone injection may be called for.
- Try both heat and cold to see which best treats your symptoms.
- Unlike tendon rupture, tendinitis will likely resolve itself, but you should follow a prescribed course of exercise to strengthen the quadriceps muscle and thus prevent a recurrence. Further weakening of the tendon from recurring tendinitis might lead to rupture in extreme cases.
- Be sure to reexamine how you perform the activity that originally caused the injury, and change your method, to avoid reinjury.

Bursitis (Housemaid's Knee)

Long-term success in treating bursitis is linked to your ability to cease or alter the activities that trigger an outbreak.

- Cease any activity that causes the irritation.
- Try a course of ice, rest, and immobilization (with an elastic bandage) to alleviate immediate symptoms.

- Your doctor may prescribe a course of NSAIDs for you.
- The doctor may aspirate your knee.
- If the inflammation persists, you may be given a steroid injection.
- Alter the triggers for your bursitis (for example, use knee pads for activities that require kneeling or instead sit on a low stool) to keep it from becoming a chronic condition.

Iliotibial Band Syndrome

- Reduce your activity, apply ice, and follow a prescribed course of muscle-strengthening exercise. These generally are all the treatment needed.
- If you have only one or two painful hot spots, a steroid injection may quiet the inflammation.
- In extreme cases, surgery may be recommended. If so, the tendon is split so that it no longer stretches tightly over the bone.

Osgood-Schlatter Disease

- Decrease the amount of activity you do, to diminish your symptoms immediately. Limit your participation in vigorous sports. Osgood-Schlatter disease generally resolves without aggressive treatment. However, alleviation of persistent symptoms may be called for.
- Apply ice to reduce the pain and inflammation.
- Wear prescribed protective knee pads if you want to continue doing active sports, and choose sports that are not

highly stressful. Apply ice if necessary after the activity to inhibit pain and swelling.

- Your doctor may prescribe a course of NSAIDs.

PATHOLOGICAL CONDITIONS AND SYNDROMES

Plica Syndrome

- Reduce your activity level. This frequently resolves the problem without extensive intervention.
- Follow the RICE regimen to deal with swelling and inflammation.
- Your doctor may prescribe a course of NSAIDs for you.
- If inflammation is extreme, your doctor may give you a cortisone injection (either specifically into the plica area or generally into the knee).
- If your pain is severe and all else fails, surgery may be called for. Through quarter-inch incisions, arthroscopic instruments are inserted to cut away and remove the plica tissue. During healing, scar tissue forms. There are no known complications from not having a plica. You will be up and about almost immediately after the operation.

Osteochondritis Dissecans

- Follow the RICE protocol. If you don't stop activity, a fragment may break loose and permanently damage your knee.
- Have the doctor determine whether the bone and cartilage are simply loose or have begun to fragment.

- If there is no fragmentation, a surgeon may fix the affected area with pins or screws.
- If fragments are loose, the surgeon may scrape the cavity to reach fresh bone, add a bone graft, and fix the fragments in position. Fragments that cannot be mended are removed, and the cavity is drilled or scraped to stimulate new cartilage growth.
- After surgery, do not bear weight on the knee for six to eight weeks or until the bone graft heals.

Osteoarthritis

- Decrease exercise that directly shocks the affected knee (such as running). However, gentle exercise (such as walking) may be useful for controlling the symptoms of osteoarthritis, since motion is vital to joint health.
- Apply ice or heat or both to relieve your symptoms.
- Your doctor may prescribe a course of NSAIDs to relieve extreme discomfort, swelling, and inflammation (some individuals cannot tolerate the pain without chronic NSAID use). However, the risks inherent in long-term NSAID use suggest that these drugs be taken sparingly.
- If previous steps do not suffice, a steroid injection may be useful when pain and swelling are localized. Steroids sometimes provide long-term relief.
- Your doctor may prescribe a hyaluronic acid injection (Hyalgan or Synvysc) to lubricate the joint, reduce inflammation, and decrease pain. (The effects may last four to six months.)
- The doctor may lavage saline into and out of the joint to wash out any small particles causing inflammation.

- Arthroscopy may be used to smooth out rough surfaces.
- If your cartilage is severely damaged, your physician may recommend cartilage replacement surgery, by either mosaicplasty or autogenous chondrocyte transplant.
- If your pain and loss of mobility are extreme, joint replacement (arthroplasty) is an option.

Rheumatoid Arthritis

Rheumatoid arthritis can be managed but not cured. It needs to be carefully monitored, because it can leave you vulnerable to fever, infection, pneumonia, and cardiovascular problems. Getting plenty of rest is vital to improving your condition, and calcium supplements are indicated to combat osteoporosis, especially if you take oral steroids regularly.

- Follow the RICE regimen.
- Undergo prescribed physical therapy.
- Your doctor may prescribe a course of NSAIDs.
- Your doctor may prescribe a course of disease-modifying antirheumatic drugs (DMARDs). These drugs come in varying strengths and are generally escalated slowly, because DMARDs can have serious side effects.
- Your doctor may recommend corticosteroid treatment, usually by injection. Steroids may also be taken orally, but that route carries far more risks than injections do. Risks associated with oral intake include osteoporosis, Cushing's syndrome, and compromise of the immune system.
- Arthroscopic or open surgery may be required to clean bone and cartilage fragments from the inflamed joint or to restructure a damaged joint.

- In severe cases, a synovectomy may be performed. Synovectomy is a surgical procedure to remove the diseased joint lining (synovial tissue) where rheumatoid arthritis originates.
- Should your joint deterioration result in extreme pain, immobility, or deformity, either arthroplasty (joint replacement) or arthrodesis (joint fusion) may be recommended, depending on your general health.

Infectious (Septic) Arthritis

- At the initial symptoms of infectious arthritis, immediately go to the doctor or emergency room.
- The doctor may aspirate your knee to remove fluid pressure and pus. A culture of the fluid will dictate which antibiotic is most potent against the specific bacteria.
- The doctor will start you on a course of antibiotics. You may be admitted to the hospital for intravenous antibiotics, which are much more effective than those taken by mouth.
- If aspiration did not adequately drain the affected area, arthroscopic surgery may be required for draining.
- You may be given analgesics as adjunct therapy.
- The joint will be immobilized until the acute phase resolves.

Chondromalacia Patellae

- Follow the RICE protocol.
- Follow a prescribed regimen of exercise and electrical muscle stimulation to strengthen the surrounding muscles. This will inhibit shifting of the patella and further roughening of the cartilage surface.

- If the symptoms resist physical therapy, you may undergo a course of NSAIDs.
- Although the results are not promising, arthroscopy may be performed to smooth the cartilage and "wash out" small fragments that can cause the knee joint to catch while bending and straightening.
- In severe cases, your surgeon may attempt to correct the angle of the kneecap by making an incision in the tendon. Cartilage removal and repositioning of misaligned structures in the knee may also be done in the procedure.

Gout

The extreme pain of a gout attack requires immediate treatment. Unfortunately, gout is not curable, and 62 percent of those who experience their first gout attack will have a second within the year.

- Follow the RICE regimen.
- You may be given a very strong NSAID, indomethacin, to relieve inflammation and pain, along with colchicine to stop inflammation.
- To provide immediate relief for the swelling and pain typical of an acute gout attack, your doctor may aspirate your knee with a syringe.
- The doctor may prescribe corticosteroids either orally or by injection.
- Follow prescribed dietary restrictions and stop your consumption of alcohol. Alcohol may have a dangerous interaction with NSAIDs. Weight loss and avoidance of certain foods can greatly reduce the likelihood and frequency of

gout attacks. These are vital components of treatment (see chapter 3).

Once repair of your knee has been accomplished, you need to undertake the hard work of completely healing the knee—and preventing future injury. Now is the time to consider knee rehabilitation.

Chapter Seven

Rehabilitating the Knee

You have completed the stages of wondering what could be wrong with your knee and then worrying whether you've made the right treatment choice. Now, in the stage of rehabilitating your knee, *you are in charge*. Doctors and rehabilitation specialists may prescribe, but acting on their recommendations is up to you. Of course, that could also be the bad news, if you're not bound and determined to do what you must do to heal.

If you don't follow the proper rehabilitation protocol, you could find yourself right back where you started, or worse, with a weak and stiff immobile knee.

This chapter examines some of the tools you'll use to help you on the road to recovery and then presents the rehabilitative therapies particular to each knee problem. Some of the protocols and information have been adapted from *Clinical Orthopedic Rehabilitation* by S. Brent Brotzman. Much of the information in this chapter I developed with my friend and colleague Dr. Gary Brazina, one of the finest and most caring of orthopedists.

BRACING THE KNEE

Knee bracing ranges from restrictive, long-legged braces that prohibit movement to simple straps that facilitate it. Braces are categorized by function as rehabilitative, functional, prophylactic, or transitional.

Rehabilitative Braces

Rehabilitative braces are used during the acute or initial phase after injury or surgery. To maintain stability, they are usually long legged and have adjustable hinges that limit motion to a specific degree. They give maximum support and allow minimum freedom of motion. They may limit the amount of knee flexion or knee extension or both. These braces are used for a short time in the postoperative or postinjury period.

Functional Braces

Functional braces control rotation of the knee and typically are used for sports activities to stabilize an unstable knee. Athletes who have had significant knee injuries use them to return to sports early while still protecting their knees. The braces are usually custom-made of light materials, such as titanium, but, because these materials cost about $1,000 per brace, generally only affluent patients or those whose insurance will cover the cost can afford functional braces.

Functional braces can be used before or after surgery. Patients who have decided not to undergo an ACL reconstruction may use a functional brace to return to some level of activity and often perform well. After ACL reconstruction, the brace may be used to protect the repair. However, a functional brace is not as restrictive as a rehabilitative brace.

Many functional bracing designs have been developed, all with advantages and disadvantages. The biggest disadvantage is that the brace may slip out of its initial position when used by a vigorous athlete, such as a skier or basketball player. The brace then causes discomfort and limits the mobility or speed the athlete needs for top performance.

Some functional braces, particularly the patellar-supporting type, are much less restrictive than others, since their main purpose is to keep the patella from slipping, tilting, or subluxing (partially dislocating). This version is useful during rehabilitation of patellofemoral syndrome.

McConnell taping can be used alone or in combination with a patellar brace. Taping has a disadvantage because it applies uncomfortable traction to the skin, which some patients find hard to tolerate. However, to stabilize a dislocating patella, a lateral buttress needs to be placed on the side of the brace.

Prophylactic Braces

Prophylactic braces are used to prevent injury to the knee. The most common type has a lateral post with two straps, one going around the tibia and one going around the femur. Bracing the outside of the knee was thought to minimize tears of the MCL, but several studies show that it actually increases the risk of injury because it puts an extra load on the medial side of the knee. Injuries may also occur with this brace because athletes feel they are protected when in fact they are not (sometimes called "the kamikaze syndrome").

Instead of using prophylactic bracing to protect your knees, try making changes in your playing surface and the type of shoes you wear. For example, use soccer-style spikes rather than the long football spikes that tend to anchor your feet in place when your body moves, forcing your knees into excess rotation.

Transitional Braces

Transitional braces are less restrictive than rehabilitative braces and often are converted versions of rehabilitative devices. They may be used after rehabilitative and before functional braces, but they are used sparingly for a variety of reasons. First, they are expensive, and insurance companies are hesitant to pay for more than two braces per patient (usually rehabilitative and functional). Second, leg girth generally increases greatly during the rehabilitative process, as muscle mass and strength are restored. A transitional brace is much more difficult to fit to accommodate the change in girth than a functional brace is.

ORTHOTICS

Gait (the way the legs and feet move while walking) plays a vital role in knee health (see chapter 1). If you have an irregular gait, orthotics may be used to correct it. Orthotics are devices inserted into shoes, and they are often used (1) to adjust the position of the standing foot, for example, if it rolls too far outward (supination) or inward (pronation) while walking; and (2) to adjust irregularities in the arch, either high arches or flat-footedness.

Orthotics range from simple over-the-counter purchases to complex and expensive pieces designed specifically for you. Whichever you use, first obtain the advice of a specialist. An orthopedist, sports rehabilitation specialist, or chiropractor is versed in gait problems and corrections.

Excess Q-angle (discussed in chapter 1), more common in females and runners, can often be prevented by correcting the pronation and supination of the foot. Changing foot mechanics with orthotics can correct misalignment of the tibia, femur, and patella.

The most common types of orthotics are the following:

- Insoles (over-the-counter orthotics) are flat, cushioned inserts designed to reduce shock, provide heel and arch support, and resist foot moisture and odor. They are successfully used by 70 percent of those with foot and gait-related problems.

• Custom-made orthotic inserts come in three forms: rigid devices, which are generally used for excessive pronation; semirigid ones, which are used primarily by athletes; and soft, cushioning inserts, which are particularly helpful for people suffering from diabetes or arthritis.

CRUTCHES AND CANES

Crutches are support devices that permit mobility when you can put little or no weight on an injured leg that is in either a brace or a cast. A cane may be used for support either temporarily, when you are regaining full mobility, or regularly, if you have permanent mobility problems. You might use a cane when you do not need a fully immobilizing brace or cast, although you do need an elastic bandage.

These rehabilitative tools are used with physical therapy and exercise to help you restore knee health.

REHABILITATIVE EXERCISES

Whether you have had surgery or not, restoring knee function is accomplished through physical rehabilitation in the form of strength and weight-bearing exercises. Always check with your doctor prior to initiating a knee exercise program. This book can educate you about the types of exercises that may help your injured knee, but it is a poor substitute for an expert who has actually seen your knee.

I think of rehabilitation as a "layer cake": The base layer, or starting point for all rehabilitation, is relief of pain, swelling, and irritation. The next layer is increasing range of motion. The third layer is strengthening. The fourth layer is a functional program, and the top layer is sport-specific training. The icing on the cake is your education about what you can or can't do, what your limitations will be, and how to manage your knee problem day to day. For example, whether your problem is chronic or acute, you need to warm your knees before exercise (perhaps by immersion in a whirlpool bath or by walking a quarter of a mile before starting to jog) and then stretch; applying cold after exercise is another excellent prescription.

Each layer of the cake is dependent on the icing covering the entire cake—your education. After total knee replacement, you must understand what sports and activities will allow your prosthetic knee to last as many years as possible. The more stress, the faster the knee will wear out, cause pain, and require surgical revision. If you are a professional athlete, you need to know how to rehabilitate quickly. The fastest way for a sports doctor to lose your confidence is to tell you to stop doing athletics. You need alternatives that can keep you active and in shape, so that you can return quickly to your sport. The best method is cross-training (exercises different from the movements of the sport that caused the injury). If you are a runner, for example, your doctor may prescribe running in a pool or weight training. These exercises allow you to maintain muscle mass and aerobic fitness, so that when your injury heals you are immediately ready to attack your sport of choice.

Keep in mind that the way you performed an activity may have caused the injury, and if so you need to correct your technique. An example is tennis elbow. Often it occurs if you hit backhand shots with your elbow bent and snapping at the ball rather than straight and driving the ball. Although bad habits are difficult to change, they can be corrected with specific drills.

Flexion of the injured or postoperative knee usually occurs easily, but extension may be difficult. The loss of full extension can lead to chronic backache. You need only 60 degrees of knee flexion to climb stairs, and there is very little you cannot do if your knee can flex to 100 degrees. An extremely effective exercise to gain full extension of the injured or postoperative knee is to walk backward slowly on a treadmill that is elevated 6 to 7 degrees.

When you rehabilitate the knee, your exercises must be specific to the injury you are healing. Consider whether you are dealing with an acute problem (a sprain of the knee, a tear of the ACL, or a tear of the meniscus, for example) or a chronic problem (such as osteoarthritis). Whether you have had surgery or not, rehabilitation is necessary.

Rehabilitative (weight-training) exercises fall into two broad categories: closed kinetic chain (CKC) exercises and open kinetic chain (OKC) exercises. A third category of exercises, aerobic exercises, uses large muscle groups repetitively for twenty to sixty minutes with the goal of increasing the maximum transport of oxygen in the body. Examples are running, spinning, biking, swimming, stair-stepping, and fast walking. Weight-training exercises produce little change in oxygen transport unless you do them with relatively light weights and do not rest between repetitions.

Isometric exercises—those that involve no movement but instead a brief tensing of muscle either alone or against an object or surface—can be either CKC or OKC. They are always a safe way to start any rehabilitation program. An example is the straight leg lift performed lying on your back (described later in this chapter). You may be surprised by how much muscle tone you can gain from this exercise when repeated frequently. Exercise protocols should also include stretching.

Closed Kinetic Chain (CKC) Exercises

Closed kinetic chain exercises are used to minimize stress across the knee joint. They require that the foot touch the floor or another object (such as in a leg press). CKC programs were developed for rehabilitation of ACL injuries, when doctors found that OKC exercises, such as leg extensions, in which the foot is free, put tremendous stress on the ACL and resulted in poor healing. We now know that it is the last 30 degrees of OKC extension that places the most stress on the ACL. This is because the ACL is at its maximum tension when the knee is fully extended, and the full range makes the knee a fulcrum with a long lever arm and increased shearing stress.

When the foot is anchored, it becomes the fulcrum, and there is less stress across the knee. CKC rather than OKC exercises are used initially after surgery or injury. Examples of rehabilitative CKC exercises are leg presses, mini-squats, stationary bicycling, and running in a pool (the foot is anchored at the point when stress is put on the knee). Squats can be dangerous if lower than 30 degrees, or if the knees are not kept over the toes. When the toes are behind the knee you increase the pressure of the patella on the femur.

Isometric Squat Stand with your knees apart. Drop down slowly to flex your hips and knees 10 degrees, keeping your knees over your toes. Rise to the starting point. Repeat, dropping another 10 degrees to 20 and then a third time to 30 degrees. Repeat the sequence ten times. Caution: Do not dip any farther or you can put strain on your knees.

Single-Leg Squat Standing with your healthy leg bent behind and off the floor, slowly drop down on your standing leg, keeping your knee over your toes, to a hip and knee flexion of 30 degrees. After an injury, you may need to hold on to something; as you recover, do the squat without holding on. Repeat ten times for one leg. Switch legs.

Step-Up Using a step (or a thick book or other substitute), tighten the quadriceps of one leg, and step up. Pull the other leg up (don't push off), then lower the leg, and step down again. Repeat ten times for one leg. Switch legs.

Side Step-Up Stand with your side facing a step. Tighten the quadriceps on the leg next to the step, and step up sideways. Pull the other leg up (don't push off), lower it, and then slowly step down. Repeat ten times for one leg. Switch legs.

Step-Down Stand with both feet on a step. Slowly lower your healthy leg to the floor (keep the injured leg on the step). Return slowly to the starting position. Repeat ten times for one leg. Switch legs.

Thigh Squeeze Stand with your back to a wall, your lower body 1 foot from the wall, and a soccer or beach ball held between your knees. Tighten your thigh muscles, and squeeze the ball. Hold for a count of twenty. Release. Repeat ten times.

Open Kinetic Chain (OKC) Exercises

OKC exercises are used earlier for chronic knee problems than for acute or postsurgical rehabilitation, but the arc of the OKC exercises is controlled. It is best to limit range of motion in OKC exercises from 30 degrees to 0 degrees (full extension) and from 90 degrees to 45 degrees, rather than the entire arc. Later in postoperative rehabilitation, OKC exercises are used more freely.

Leg Lift Lie faceup on the floor. If your knee is injured, keep that leg straight during the exercise (otherwise, in this and all exercises, alternate your legs for strengthening). Bend the healthy knee to a 90-degree angle, foot on the floor. Lift the straight leg up until it is as high as the bent knee. Hold for a count of three. Lower. Repeat ten times for one leg.

Side Leg Lift Lie faceup on floor. Bend the healthy knee to a 90-degree angle, foot on the floor. Extend the injured leg, and roll that foot to the side so that the inner side of the knee faces upward. Lift the rolled leg 1 to 2 feet above the floor, hold for a count of three, and lower slowly. Repeat ten times for one leg. If both legs are healthy, alternate after ten lifts.

Bent Side Leg Lift Lie faceup on floor. Bend the healthy knee to 90 degrees, foot on the floor. Extend the injured leg, roll that foot to the side so that inside of the knee faces upward, and then bend that knee slightly. Lift the rolled leg 8 to 12 inches, hold for a count of three, and lower it. Repeat ten times for one leg. If both legs are healthy, alternate after ten repetitions.

Thigh Tightener—Quadriceps (Isometric) Lie faceup on the floor, injured leg straight, healthy knee bent 90 degrees, foot on the floor. Contract the straight leg muscles, trying to push the back of your knee against the floor. Hold for a count of three. Repeat ten times for one leg.

Thigh Tightener—Hamstring (Isometric) Lie faceup on the floor, injured leg straight, healthy knee bent 90 degrees, foot on the floor. Push the heel of your straight leg into floor. Hold for a count of three. Repeat ten times for one leg.

Kneecap Bounce You can perform this exercise anywhere. Doing it daily—at your desk, at home in a chair, or while waiting on line—can greatly improve your knee health. (It is a closed kinetic chain exercise if you keep your foot on the floor.) While standing or sitting, straighten the injured leg, contract the knee muscles for one to five seconds, and then release. During the contraction phase, the kneecap will bounce. Repeat at least ten times and as many as you can tolerate.

Aerobic Exercise

You may need to halt or limit some aerobic activities during knee recovery. In Exhibit 7.1, I offer two lists of activities that may be beneficial at some point during your rehabilitation: (1) an acceptable activities list, which indicates pursuits that are unlikely to cause problems if you have not had a major injury and do not have a pain-causing syndrome; and (2) a problematic activities list, which contains activities that also may be beneficial but that you should not attempt without counsel and approval from your physician or physical therapist (who generally is in consultation with your doctor).

PROTOCOLS FOR SPECIFIC INJURIES

It is mandatory that you check with your physician before following any of these exercise programs. Your injury and health status are unique.

As you go through the following protocols, keep in mind that the length and complexity of the protocol vary with the severity and complexity of the knee injury. For that reason, some protocols are more detailed (week by week) while others give only general long-term exercises. Even when a weekly schedule is described, gaps may be left in the timetable because individuals vary in their progress.

No protocol here should be seen as an absolute; rather it is merely a likely outline of the specific plan your physician will prescribe for you.

Anterior Cruciate Ligament (ACL) Injury

Rehabilitation for ACL injuries begins even before surgery is performed. There is controversy among experts about how quickly

EXHIBIT 7.1 Acceptable and Problematic Activities
During Rehabilitation

Acceptable Activities and
Exercise Equipment

- Fast walking
- Water aerobics
- Swimming (crawl stroke, flutter kick)
- Cross-country ski glide machine
- Walking on soft-platform treadmill
- Trampoline

Problematic Activities and
Exercise Equipment

- Squatting
- Kneeling
- Twisting and pivoting
- Repetitive bending (such as stair climbing)
- Jogging
- Jazzercize
- Racquetball
- Tennis
- Basketball
- Swimming (frog or whip kick)
- Bicycling
- Stair-step machine
- Stationary bicycle
- Rowing machine
- Leg extension weight machine
- Power yoga

surgery should be undertaken, and some studies show that waiting several weeks before surgery yields a quicker return of full range of motion (ROM) after surgery.

Waiting requires rehabilitation both preoperatively and for nine months postoperatively, however, and many patients would rather just have the surgery done quickly.

Preoperative Protocol Preoperative therapy concentrates on reducing the pain and swelling and attempting full ROM. Decreasing joint effusion is key to all these goals. It is done through compression, elevation, cryotherapy (application of cold), and electrical stimulation. If all else fails, your knee may be aspirated by syringe.

Inhibiting joint effusion is vital if you are to restore ROM and inhibit atrophy of the quadriceps muscle. A six-week rehabilitation program before surgery allows you to build good quadriceps and hamstring strength. If your knee responds well, surgery may not be needed. Even if surgery is necessary, your postoperative rehabilitation program will be easier with well-toned muscles, and your likelihood of full recovery will be greatly improved.

Postoperative Protocol During the first week after surgery, rehabilitation is mostly passive. Your leg may be placed in a continuous passive motion (CPM) machine for many hours a day to gently increase its range of motion. CPM assists patellar mobility and reduces scarring of the patella. Regular icing and elevation are used to reduce swelling. Your goal is full extension (or 10 degrees short of that) and 70 degrees of flexion by the end of the first week.

By week two you begin gait training so that you are comfortable with full weight-bearing and comfortable with crutches. If strong enough, you can walk without the crutches but using a brace. You begin isometric exercises and slowly increase your ROM. As soon as the swelling is controlled, you can use a stationary bike and can start gluteal strengthening exercises to stabilize your pelvis. These exercises include isometric pushes of the leg against a wall and inner and outer thigh exercises with a ball. Balancing on either foot stimulates isometric toning of the quadriceps and hamstrings and helps reestablish proprioception (ability to know where your leg is), which is diminished after an ACL tear.

By week three, you begin more active quadriceps strengthening with increased range of motion, using a Thera-Band or a sport cord on both the uninjured and the injured leg. The uninjured leg is strengthened to increase pelvic stability.

Walking in water, running in a pool, and walking backward on a treadmill are excellent exercises at this stage. Nonimpact reciprocal or elliptical trainers can be used to strengthen your muscles and maintain your aerobic capacity. You can use the leg press and balance board and do hamstring strengthening exercises. At four to six weeks, start using a cross-country ski machine, such as the Nordic Track.

At about eight weeks, focus on your proprioception and coordination by stepping forward, stepping backward, and balancing on a slide board. Add stair climbing on the StairMaster, both forward and backward.

By the third to fourth month, you can begin running figure eights. Although you are not allowed to participate in vigorous sports for at least six and preferably nine months, you can mimic the movements of the sport you love. If it's tennis, for example, begin to move forward to back and side to side, with stops and starts. After four months you can attempt pliometrics (jumping and explosive types of training).

A functional brace is generally recommended for sports activity for at least the first year after surgery. Be warned that a knee without pain is not an indication that your ACL is completely recovered. ACLs are not totally healed (the graft isn't fully mature) until about nine months after surgery. Many ACLs are reinjured because patients resume sports activities too soon.

Medial and Lateral Collateral Ligament Injuries

MCL and LCL injuries come in three grades: Grades one and two are partial tears of varying degrees, while grade three is a complete tear. Unless accompanied by other ligament tears, MCL and LCL injuries are generally treated without surgery.

Lower-grade injuries are milder than higher-grade ones and require less rehabilitation. The protocol is similar to that for ACL injury (preoperative and postoperative), described in the preceding section, but the time required for healing is shorter—usually only four to six weeks—because you do not need to wait for a tendon graft to mature.

Posterior Cruciate Ligament (PCL) Injury

PCL tears rarely require surgery but the rehabilitation protocol is the same as for ACL injuries (preoperative and postoperative), described earlier. The only major difference is that the posterior cruciate ligament is at maximum stress across the knee when it is flexed. Therefore extension exercises are emphasized more than flexion exercises.

Meniscal Injury

Depending on its severity, a meniscal injury may or may not require surgery. When the tear is minor, after your pain and other symptoms abate, your physician may prescribe a course of exercises. If no surgery is needed, once the swelling has subsided, you can move rapidly into resistance exercises.

If surgery is called for, one of two procedures will be done: suturing of the meniscal tear or, in extreme injuries, full or partial removal of the meniscus. One goal of rehabilitation is to protect weight loading of the knee, especially loading in flexion, until at least six to eight weeks postoperatively. CKC exercises are started early, with flexion limited to 70 to 80 degrees. OKC exercises are avoided until at least six months after a meniscal repair. Starting to move as early as possible after surgery is critical.

Dislocation of the Patella

Dislocation of the patella is an extremely painful, traumatic, and quite common injury. It requires careful rehabilitation. Some experts advocate surgical repair of the first dislocation to prevent subsequent ones that can damage the undersurface of the patella and the femoral track. Other experts advise waiting until the second or third dislocation before doing a surgical repair.

When the injury is acute, your knee will be immobilized in a brace that keeps it in extension and limits flexion. After full extension for about two weeks, you slowly increase flexion for about six weeks. You concentrate on terminal arc extension, strengthening the vastus medialis oblique muscle, and stretching the vastus lateralis. Patellar taping (McConnell taping) is helpful at this stage. Then your injury may be treated conservatively by muscle retraining and use of orthotics, or surgical intervention may be necessary. Stationary biking and walking backward on a treadmill are great exercises for dislocation recovery.

Rupture of the Patellar Tendon

Rupture of the patellar tendon is treated either by immobilization in a cast, if the doctor believes the rupture will heal by scarring, or by surgical repair. The rehabilitation protocol follows that for patellar dislocation (described in the preceding section), tailored individually according to how your healing is progressing.

Fracture

The key to recovery after a fracture is for the physician to align the bone as perfectly as is humanly possible. Postoperatively you keep weight off the leg for at least six weeks, but you begin active ROM exercises early. Once the fracture has healed, you follow a traditional program of CKC strengthening exercises. Use pool therapy first by actively swishing the leg through the water and, after healing, by running in the pool. Postpone a strengthening program until the fracture is solid.

Stress Fracture

When you experience a stress fracture, stop the activity that caused it (often running), and change the sport. It takes about six weeks for the fracture to heal. Use alternatives to running, such as stationary biking and running in a pool.

Patellofemoral Syndrome (Runner's Knee)

Runner's knee generally describes a kneecap that slips and catches, most often because the vastus medialis oblique muscle, which is primarily charged with keeping the patella in its proper place, has been weakened. Rehabilitation generally takes six weeks. Exercises are not done on a timetable but rather based on your own judgment and tolerance.

Exercises to avoid when you have this syndrome include step classes, high impact aerobics, cycling, hill cycling, and hill running. Cycling on a flat course is good if you don't rise off your seat. One of the most common causes of this syndrome is cycling with the seat too low and using too high a gear. These factors cause the patella to be jammed too deeply into the femoral groove. People who do deep squats are also at risk for patellofemoral syndrome.

Tendinitis

To reduce pain and inflammation and to strengthen the quadriceps muscles, which can prevent a recurrence of the injury, follow the course of exercise described later in this chapter for osteoarthritis rehabilitation after nonsurgical treatment. Focus on strengthening the muscles connected to the patellar tendon, which will relieve strain on the tendon. Take care not to return too quickly to exercises that stress the area. You need to recover fully and avoid a relapse.

Bursitis (Housemaid's Knee)

Follow the exercises described later in this chapter for osteoarthritis rehabilitation after nonsurgical treatment, to strengthen the knee.

Iliotibial Band Syndrome

Follow a prescribed course of exercise to stretch the iliotibial band. Insert a lateral heel wedge in your shoe, and wear soft running shoes rather than hard shoes. Once you resume activity, only slowly attempt running downhill and on pitched surfaces and for only short episodes.

Osgood-Schlatter Disease

Follow the exercises described later in this chapter for osteoarthritis rehabilitation after nonsurgical treatment.

Plica Syndrome

After reducing your activity level to deal with inflammation, begin minimal ROM rehabilitation exercises. When you achieve satisfactory ROM, you can initiate all activities as tolerated.

Osteochondritis Dissecans

Rehabilitation for osteochondritis dissecans is similar to that for a fracture. Keep weight off the leg for six weeks, but initiate ROM exercises early. Then follow the exercises described later in this chapter for osteoarthritis rehabilitation after nonsurgical treatment.

Osteoarthritis

The rehabilitation protocol for the osteoarthritic knee depends on the severity of the treatment you have undergone.

Nonsurgical Treatment If you have experienced pain, some stiffness, and swelling in the knee but your mobility in general is unaffected, the following course is prescribed for rehabilitating osteoarthritis and minimizing further damage to the joint. In addition, if you are overweight, any weight loss is beneficial because it reduces stress on the knee.

Wear prescribed inserts to cushion against knee shock, and eliminate activities that shock the joint (such as running and racquetball). Begin gentle exercise (such as walking) to "feed" the joint, inhibit joint stiffness, and prevent tissue atrophy. To help safeguard your knee by creating stronger support for the joint and inhibiting excessive movement and friction that can cause irritation, perform muscle- and strength-building exercises, such as leg lifts, stationary bicycling (for 20 to 60 minutes), isometric squats with your back against a wall (held for 60 seconds), and running in water up to your chest.

Arthroscopic Surgical Treatment If you undergo arthroscopy, you usually are released from the hospital right away but asked to stay off your feet for three to four days. Early ROM and strengthening exercise protocols are prescribed depending on the type of surgery performed.

Surgical Joint Replacement Rehabilitation after a joint replacement may be quite lengthy, depending upon both the surgeon's skill and your general condition. You should expect to spend a week in the hospital after surgery, because your bones have been cut to receive the prosthesis. Early ROM and strengthening exercise protocols are critical to rehabilitation.

Use crutches for two to four weeks after surgery. If possible, begin physical therapy three days after surgery. Studies have shown that this results in a far quicker recovery than waiting a week (which used to be the common practice).

In the first month, perform OKC and CKC exercises. After three months, you should be able to walk several miles and safely climb stairs, although running is still prohibited. Your final ROM will generally not exceed 110 degrees.

Rheumatoid Arthritis

Follow the exercises described earlier in this chapter for osteoarthritis rehabilitation after nonsurgical treatment.

Infectious (Septic) Arthritis

After the acute infection subsides, a therapist will manipulate your joint in passive ROM exercises; as your pain diminishes, perform weight-bearing CKC and OKC exercises as tolerated to restore your strength and stability.

Chondromalacia Patellae

After your pain subsides, follow the exercises described earlier in this chapter for osteoarthritis rehabilitation after nonsurgical treatment, as tolerated.

Gout

After the pain of an acute episode resolves, follow the exercises described earlier in this chapter for osteoarthritis rehabilitation after nonsurgical treatment, as tolerated.

Chapter Eight

Alternative Healing and the Knee

■■■■■■■

Although there is a huge gap between traditional Western medicine and alternative medicine, many practitioners now integrate both methods in their practice. The strange thing about alternative medicine is that many years ago, before the advent of high technology, it was the traditional practice. Take a look at an old *Merck Manual*. It contains much of what is now considered alternative medicine.

Thanks to the efforts of nutritional pioneers such as Adele Davis and Dr. Robert Atkins and the work of best-selling authors like Dr. Andrew Weil, Dr. Deepak Chopra, Dr. John Sarno, and Dr. Dean Ornish, people increasingly look to combine the benefits of Eastern medicine, homeopathy, and other alternative treatments with those of traditional medicine. This chapter discusses how alternative practices might be useful for both healing the knee and reducing pain in chronic knee problems.

ACUPRESSURE

Acupressure seeks to remedy illness by applying deep finger pressure at specific points throughout the body. It may be effective for relieving headache, muscle and joint aches, and tension and for promoting relaxation. The Japanese version of acupressure is shiatsu; *tuina* is a Chinese variation of the same practice.

ACUPUNCTURE

Originating in China more than five thousand years ago, acupuncture is founded on the belief that health requires a balanced flow of *chi*—the vital life force present in all living organisms. Acupuncture balances the body by inserting needles at points on the body specific to the problem. It works to "tonify" or sedate either *yin* or *yang*, the two opposite and complementary forces in the world, and to correct and rebalance energy flow, relieving pain and restoring health.

In terms of knee problems, acupuncture has been shown to have great benefits for those suffering from osteoarthritis and rheumatoid arthritis, knee trauma, and overuse syndromes. Studies have also shown that acupuncture stimulates the release of endorphins and enkephalins, the body's natural painkilling chemicals. Acupuncture thus literally alters your perception of pain and offers pain relief. In practice, patients commonly watch knee swelling and bruising diminish within a few hours after a session of needling.

The book *Medical Acupuncture* by Joseph Helms, M.D., of UCLA (the leading guru of acupuncture for medical doctors), discusses and illustrates the acupuncture points specific for healing the knee.

AYURVEDIC MEDICINE

Ayurvedic medicine is not a specific treatment but instead an East Indian medical system that has been practiced for more than two thousand years. The goal of Ayurvedic medicine is to prevent disease by balancing your *dosha*, or metabolic type. There are three primary *dosha* categories: *kapha*, the calm, somewhat lethargic, and over-weight people who need coffee to get started and may lie in bed when depressed; *pitta*, the competitive, quick-tempered people; and *vata*, the thin, quick, energetic mentalizers who often have difficulty sleeping. These types compare somewhat to the Western categories of endomorphs, mesomorphs, and ectomorphs. Bringing these *dosha* into balance is done through a combination of diet, herbs, laxatives, massage, stretching, breathing exercises, and yoga.

If your knee problems are related to arthritis, you may find some relief from a plant extract formulation called RA-1 that is used in Ayurvedic medicine. A randomized trial, with results published in the *Journal of Rheumatology* (June 2000), found that subjects using RA-1 showed a modest improvement in pain and swelling over those using a placebo.

Dr. Arvind Chopra of the Bharati Hospital Medical College in Pune, India, reported that, in a three-year follow-up study with an increased dosage of RA-1, 40 percent of patients found significant relief from regular use of the herbal remedy. Sponsorship for comparative drug trials is currently being sought.

CHIROPRACTIC MEDICINE

Chiropractic is a branch of the healing arts that is based on the understanding that good health depends in part on a normally functioning nervous system (especially the spine and the nerves extending from the spine to all parts of the body).

Chiropractic comes from the Greek word *chiropraktikos*, meaning "effective treatment by hand." Chiropractors locate and adjust musculoskeletal areas of the body which function improperly and restore normal function to the muscles, joints, and nerves. Doctors of chiropractic use the time-honored methods of consultation, case history, physical examination, and X-ray examination.

Chiropractic is synergistic with all other healing modalities. It assists in realigning the body, while other modalities are taking effect.

The spine is not the only body part that chiropractors adjust. Frequently, an adjustment to the knee will stop pain and reduce inflammation. Chiropractors may also reduce knee pain by adjusting the mechanics of gait with braces and orthotics. In addition, they are experts in knee nutrition.

HERBAL MEDICINE

Although you may think of herbal remedies as an old-fashioned or "New Age" alternative, the truth is that 25 percent of all prescription drugs are based on herbs and 74 percent of those use herbs in the same way that native cultures used them as plant medicines.

Interest in herbal medicine has greatly increased in recent years. Pharmaceutical companies haven't promoted the use of herbs, because herbs can't be patented, and this greatly limits the revenue to be gained from them. However, the federal Dietary Supplement Health and Education Act of 1994 eased Federal Drug Administration restrictions on herbs and all natural, nondrug supplements. Consequently, mainstream distributors such as One A Day have created their own lines of herbal supplements, and these have stimulated public interest and awareness.

Herbs may or may not offer the same rapid relief as pharmaceutical drugs, but when properly administered they may offer a healthful, gentle way to relieve a number of conditions.

For knee problems, anti-inflammatory herbs may be an excellent alternative to drugs, particularly for treating chronic conditions, because long-term use of NSAIDs can damage the stomach, kidneys, and liver. By taking a whole-body approach, focusing not just on relief of your pain but also on the health of all your organs, you simultaneously reduce your symptoms of swelling, reduce the resultant pain, and reduce the stomach irritation and other problems related to traditional anti-inflammatories. An herbal anti-inflammatory such as Saint-John's-wort, which has mild pain-relieving and sedative properties, can also help ease the depression that accompanies chronic physical problems. Kava kava (from the plant *Piper methysticum*) may also be useful to reduce pain-driven anxiety.

HYPNOTHERAPY

Hypnotherapy is primarily used to control and relieve long-term (chronic) pain. At minimum, hypnosis can put patients into a relaxed state that pain may have kept them from achieving. At maximum, hypnosis has enabled patients who are completely intolerant of traditional anesthetics to undergo surgery without anesthesia.

Hypnotherapy may help you deal with pain related to physical injury. It may also assist the mind/body connection by uncovering anxieties, stressors, or beliefs that may be inhibiting your ability to move forward and heal.

Formally sanctioned by the American Medical Association in 1958, hypnosis is a valid and valuable tool, but only if practiced by a skilled professional. It is vital to investigate the credentials and references of any hypnotherapist you engage.

MAGNETIC FIELD THERAPY

Practitioners of magnetic field therapy believe that pain resulting from damaged or diseased tissue is a disorder of the magnetic resonance of normal atoms, molecules, cells, and tissues of the body. Magnets are used to restore these body components to their proper resonance, thereby relieving the pain.

This treatment uses a range of magnets, from the small, handheld variety, which may be affixed over the affected area by elastic bandage or Velcro, to the Magnetic Resonance Analyzer (MRA) developed by Ronald J. Weinstock. This machine first uses magnetic force to analyze the normal magnetic resonance patterns of your tissue, and then corrects any abnormalities by sending a neutralizing resonance field back into the body. A study of MRA use at the Joint Rehabilitation and Sports Medical Center in Los Angeles is showing success in reducing knee pain.

Other studies have shown that magnets effectively reduced the pain of long-term sufferers. The *Archives of Physical Medicine and Rehabilitation* (November 1997) reported that polio patients found relief from painful trigger points with the use of magnets. The group subjected to a placebo did not experience the same relief.

Magnet therapy is generally without side effects, although pregnant women or patients with a cardiac pacemaker should check with their physician prior to using this treatment.

If you suffer from long-term knee pain, magnetic field therapy may be useful for pain management and should have no ill effects on the injured knee. If other pain therapies have not brought you relief, it is certainly worth trying.

NATUROPATHY

Naturopathy encompasses a broad range of natural and noninvasive treatments, ranging from a diet high in fruits, vegetables, and fiber to more controversial "detoxifying" procedures using herbs, enemas, and hydrotherapy. While the benefits of good nutrition are widely accepted, you should exercise caution before engaging in an herbal or detoxifying regimen, because these treatments can be quite harmful if not properly administered.

Naturopathy originated in the nineteenth century as a response to the diseases and pollution resulting from the Industrial Revolution. Its advocates promoted the benefits of fresh air, sunshine, and saltwater—still good prescriptions for feeling better, as anyone who has spent a long day at the beach can attest. Naturopathy also spawned advocacy of health food, drawing proponents such as Dr. W. K. Kellogg (also famous for his cereal company), who instructed his well-to-do followers to eschew meat, exercise regularly, and give themselves enemas twice a day. The practice fell out of favor with the rise of organized medicine and advances in pharmaceutical research after World War II. It had a resurgence based on the works of nutritionist Adele Davis, vitamin C advocate Linus Pauling, and others during the 1960s and 1970s.

What can naturopathy offer those suffering with knee problems? First, the nutritious diet prescribed by naturopaths is an excellent way to pursue weight loss, and taking weight off the knee can go a long way toward reducing pain and immobility. Second, some natural remedies help relieve pain and inflammation.

However, be as cautious about working with a naturopath as with any other practitioner. "Natural" does not mean safe from the dangers of side effects and drug interactions. For example, Saint-John's-wort is an herbal antidepressant, but if you take too high a dose or take it concomitantly with a drug such as Prozac or Paxil, you could suffer serious side effects.

Naturopaths are licensed in eleven states. The most advanced are N.D.s (Doctors of Naturopathic Medicine), who have completed four years of graduate training at a naturopathic college.

NUTRITIONAL SUPPLEMENTS

The use of nutritional supplements for joint health became a topic of national discussion with the 1997 publication of *The Arthritis Cure* by Jason Theodosakis, M.D. The book discussed glucosamine and chondroitin sulfate not as actual cures but as inhibitors of the joint degeneration and pain associated with osteoarthritis.

Both glucosamine and chondroitin sulfate are building blocks of cartilage. Glucosamine is believed to stimulate the cartilage formation required for joint repair. Chondroitin sulfate is thought to maintain joint viscosity, stimulate cartilage repair mechanisms, and inhibit the enzymes that break down cartilage.

Veterinarians have long used a combination of glucosamine and chondroitin sulfate to treat arthritis in animals. Animal studies have shown that oral glucosamine supplements had benefits for reducing inflammation, mechanical arthritis, and immunological reactive arthritis, although not to the extent of drug therapies such as indomethacin, which is an NSAID.

Human trials, too, have shown positive results in pain reduction, increased mobility, and reduction of inflammation. Some studies also showed that cartilage integrity was maintained from the time patients began taking the supplements, while study subjects taking placebos experienced cartilage deterioration at the rate normally associated with osteoarthritis. However, the *Journal of American Medicine*, among others, reviewed the studies and found them deficient in several areas—length of study, number of participants, and exaggeration of claimed benefits. Despite this, however, the reviewers did not dismiss the likelihood that these supplements offer some benefits to some patients. They cautioned only that studies thus far have not offered conclusive proof that the supplements do so.

Many questions about nutritional supplements are about to be answered. The National Institutes of Health have dedicated $6.6 million to a double-blind study on the effects of glucosamine and chondroitin sulfate (both separately and in combination) versus placebos. The study will follow one thousand participants over four months and track pain levels, joint mobility, and cartilage deterioration (through X rays taken at the outset and finish of the study).

Although this study is not complete, it has not documented adverse side effects so far from taking these supplements. However, patients considering the supplements need to consider several precautions.

Some experts have raised concern that glucosamine and chondroitin may slightly raise blood-sugar levels and could therefore be a problem for the many diabetes sufferers in this country. While current evidence of this is inconclusive, if you have even a pre-diabetic condition, exercise caution, consult your doctor, and closely monitor your blood sugar levels should you pursue a course of supplementation.

Never blindly substitute nutritional supplements for prescribed medications unless advised to do so by a medical professional. The anti-inflammatory properties of the supplements may, however, reduce your dependence on NSAIDs and, as a result, reduce such side effects as stomach upset, ulcers, kidney problems, and liver problems.

Studies have shown that some brands of glucosamine and chondroitin do not contain the full strength claimed on the bottle. Generally recommended daily dosages are 1,500 mg for glucosamine and 1,200 mg for chondroitin. Choose established supplement manufacturers, and check expiration dates to avoid buying degraded product, so that you get the product—and benefits—you're paying for. The supplements are not cheap, and no insurance company will pay the cost as they will for pharmaceutical NSAIDs.

More traditionally, calcium intake is important for bone health. Supplements and dairy products are good calcium sources, but some people don't realize that dark green, leafy vegetables such as kale are phenomenal sources of easily absorbed calcium as well.

Vitamin D assists the body in calcium absorption, and its deficiency is a common problem among osteoarthritis patients. A 1996 report in the *Annals of Internal Medicine* indicated an association between the progression of osteoarthritis and low intake and blood levels of vitamin D. The report cites a study by Tim E. McAlidin, M.D., of 556 patients who averaged seventy years of age. In subjects with vitamin D deficiency, osteoarthritis progressed at a rate three times greater than in those with normal vitamin D levels.

Vitamin D supplementation is not entirely risk-free. If you take excessive dosages, your body may reabsorb calcium from your bones and deposit it in soft tissues such as the heart and lungs, possibly inhibiting their ability to function properly. Consult your physician before considering anything more than the recommended daily amount of supplementation.

PROLOTHERAPY

Prolotherapy is defined in *Webster's New Collegiate Dictionary* as "The rehabilitation of incompetent structures such as a ligament or tendon by the induced proliferation of new cells." Ligaments, the tendons, and the joint capsular tissue are made of collagen. Prolotherapy is the simple practice of stimulating the body to proliferate, or produce more, collagen naturally.

Weakness or laxness of the ligaments and tendons may lead to increased cartilage degeneration and finally bone-on-bone friction, with resultant arthritis pain. Additionally, nerves around the soft tissues become stretched and irritated, producing pain.

With prolotherapy, dextrose (sugar water) or a stronger proliferent-based solution (blood, phenol, sodium morhuate, or glycerin, or a combination) is injected with a syringe directly into the area where the affected ligament, joint capsule, or tendon attaches to the bone. This injection stimulates cell growth and results in a stronger or larger tendon or ligament that can hold body structures in place more effectively. The weakened area heals, and the patient's pain is reduced or eliminated. It is an excellent alternative to cortisone injections in the knee.

Prolotherapy's modern model was founded in the 1950s by Drs. George Hackett and Gustav Hemwall, but the notion of irritating an injured area to stimulate the body to heal itself goes back to ancient Greece. Hippocrates, the great Greek physician whom modern doctors honor when they take the Hippocratic oath, treated soldiers suffering torn and dislocated shoulders by piercing the injured area with an iron heated in a fire. As a result, the collagen in the area would shrink and a scar would form. Although modern prolotherapy entails minimal pain, as any injection does, it is certainly mild compared to that ancient practice.

Most patients require about half a dozen prolotherapy treatments to restore function and relieve pain, but many find improvement after only one session. Aside from pain caused by either the injection or possible bruising or stiffness after the treatment, few serious side effects have occurred in the tens of thousands of people successfully treated by prolotherapy. Although only a few doctors practice this nonsurgical treatment, it is heartily endorsed by former Surgeon General C. Everett Koop, who himself was a prolotherapist (see his Web site, DrKoop.com, for his prolotherapy page). Diet guru Robert Atkins, M.D., also uses "prolo" at his New York clinic and calls it a miraculous treatment.

REFLEXOLOGY

Reflexology is a treatment based upon the belief that the foot is a microcosm for the entire body and that pressure on various "reflex points" of the foot can offer relief from symptoms found elsewhere in the body. Reflexology is not designed to cure ailments but rather to relieve symptoms of a variety of stress-related syndromes, headache, chronic arthritis pain, and other conditions.

Current reflexology is based on a map of the foot that illustrates specific pressure points and the areas of the body that they affect. The first version of this chart was created in the early 1900s by Dr. William H. Fitzgerald, and the chart was refined in the 1930s by Eunice Ingham, a nurse and physiotherapist.

Although reflexology was originally thought to work in the same way as acupressure and acupuncture—by unblocking vital energy.

Although reflexology was originally thought to work in the same way as acupressure and acupuncture—by unblocking vital energy flows throughout the body—current practitioners believe that other reasons account for the treatment's success. Some think that manipulation brings benefits by reducing the amount of lactic acid in the tissues and releasing calcium crystals accumulated in the foot's nerve endings. These crystals are believed to hold back the free flow of energy to corresponding organs. Other practitioners think that pressure on the trigger points may stimulate the release of pain-neutralizing endorphins. Yet another theory is that the therapy opens blood vessels and improves circulation. Finally, some believe that reflexology has a detoxifying effect because it dissolves crystals of uric acid that settle in the feet.

A variety of patients with knee conditions may find that their symptoms are relieved through reflexology. Increased circulation and pain relief are helpful for both the postoperative patient and the osteoarthritis sufferer. Unlike knee exercises, reflexology may offer relief without compounding or aggravating an existing knee injury or condition.

Afterword

Healing occurs not just on the physical level but also on emotional, mental, and spiritual levels, what I call *healing from within*. Although patients visit me for a specific physical problem, the common denominator for us all seems to be a quest for the meaning of life, for joy in the midst of hardship and stress. Most pain flares arise during periods in our lives that are difficult in other ways, and we seem to find it easier to focus on and deal with physical issues than to explore difficulties and truths about who we really are inside. The fear we may harbor that we are not perfect just the way we are is very painful in itself and can augment physical pain we are experiencing.

Years ago, this somatization of emotional pain into physical problems tended to manifest itself in gastric ulcers. Your father probably had an ulcer, while you are instead beset with knee or other pain. I frequently see patients shift from years of depression to focus on a physical pain, which is a more socially acceptable issue. They aren't held to blame for their physical pain, whereas depression and anxiety are problems that make them "bad" people, hard to deal with or needing lots of time and care from others.

In many cases, I find that my job is to take away a patient's diagnosis. Doctors often unknowingly brand patients with diagnoses. Some patients clutch these as the central meaning of their lives, a reason to be miserable, to be victims. "I am a medial meniscus tear" is what I hear between the lines. Frequently, the given diagnosis is wrong anyway. Just because an MRI of the knee shows a meniscal tear does not mean that that is the cause of the pain. Several studies have proved that many people who were diagnosed by an MRI or other methods as having anatomic lesions do not have pain at all.

It is my sincere hope that you will continue to search for the answers to your healing as I search for mine. Look for a doctor who brings joy to your life. That's where the healing begins. Don't settle for less than you deserve.

Glossary

Acupressure A traditional Chinese healing practice that seeks to promote wellness by applying deep finger pressure at acupuncture points.

Acupuncture A traditional Chinese therapy in which thin needles are inserted into specific points in the body to inhibit pain and stress, promote healing, and bring the body into balance.

Allograft A transplant of preserved tissue or a preserved organ, harvested after the donor's death.

Anterior cruciate ligament (ACL) A ligament connecting the femur and tibia, which is found inside and to the front of the knee joint.

Arthritis Technically, inflammation of a joint; clinically, breakdown of the structures in and around a joint.

Arthrodesis The surgical procedure of fusing a joint.

Arthroplasty The surgical procedure of replacing a joint with a prosthesis (artificial body part).

Arthroscopy (arthroscopic surgery) A form of surgery in which the doctor inserts a tiny camera to see inside a joint and operates through very small incisions.

Articular cartilage The smooth cartilage covering the ends of bones, which facilitates easy gliding motion in a joint.

Aspirate To remove fluids or other matter, using a syringe.

Autogenous chondrocyte transplant A two-step surgical procedure in which cartilage cells are first cultured and then placed in damaged sections of cartilage and covered with tissue so that they can regenerate.

Autoimmune dysfunction A condition in which the body's immune system reacts to its own tissue or cell types as if they were foreign matter.

Avascular Not fed by blood; for example, cartilage is avascular.

Ayurvedic medicine An East Indian medical system designed to promote wellness by bringing a person's *dosha*, or metabolic type, into balance.

Bursa A small, fluid-filled sac that cushions the points of contact between bones, tendons, and ligaments.

Bursitis (housemaid's knee) Inflammation of one or more bursae.

Cartilage A tough, white, fibrous connective tissue found throughout the body, particularly in the joints. *See also* Articular cartilage.

Chiropractic A therapy involving balancing the body and manipulating the spine and other body structures to relieve pain and promote mobility and healing.

Chondral surface The glassy-smooth cartilage surface.

Chondral transplantation A surgical procedure to replace cartilage.

Chondroitin sulfate A building block of cartilage; it is used as a nutritional supplement to promote joint health.

Chondromalacia patellae A condition in which the articular cartilage on the back of the patella is softened or worn down.

CKC exercise *See* Closed kinetic chain exercise.

Closed kinetic chain (CKC) exercise Exercise in which the foot maintains contact with a surface. Examples are squats and bicycling.

Collagen The fibrous protein constituent of connective tissue in the body.

Computerized tomography (CT) scan An X-ray procedure that combines a number of X-ray pictures with computer enhancement to generate cross-sectional and three-dimensional images of the body's internal structures and organs.

Contracture A shortening of a muscle, tendon, or ligament, which inhibits full range of motion.

Corticosteroid A steroid hormone produced by the adrenal cortex, or its synthetic equivalent.

Cortisone An anti-inflammatory steroid commonly used in the treatment of arthritis, tendinitis, and bursitis.

Crepitus A cracking or crunching sound when the joint is moved.

CT scan *See* Computerized tomography scan.

Degenerative arthritis *See* Osteoarthritis.

Dorsiflexion Tilting of the foot upward at the ankle.

Embolus A plug in a blood vessel that travels from its source.

Etiology The underlying cause of a disease or disorder.

Femur The thighbone.

Fibula The narrow, outer bone of the lower leg.

Gait The way the legs and feet move while walking.

Gait cycle A unit of two complete walking steps.

Glucosamine sulfate A building block of cartilage; it is used as a nutritional supplement to reduce pain and promote joint health.

Gout An arthritic inflammation of a joint resulting from excess uric acid in the body.

Graft A transplant of tissue from one part of the body to another or from one body to another.

Hamstring muscles The group of muscles in back of the thigh.

Hemarthrosis An accumulation of blood in the joint.

Hyperextend To overstraighten.

Hypertrophy A condition in which muscle or bone grows beyond its normal state.

Hypnosis An induced dreamlike state that renders a person suscep-tible to suggestion and free to recall memories and details that may be blocked during full consciousness.

Hypnotherapy A treatment using hypnosis, for example to inhibit pain and stress.

Iliotibial band A thickened strip of fascia, the fibrous tissue that connects the hip to the side of the knee.

Iliotibial band syndrome An inflammatory condition of the iliotibial band resulting from overuse.

Infectious (septic) arthritis Arthritis caused by infection in a joint.

Joint effusion Fluid accumulation in a joint.

Lateral collateral ligament (LCL) The ligament attaching the femur to the fibula, which is found outside the knee on the lateral (outer) side of the leg.

Magnetic resonance imaging (MRI) A diagnostic technique in which a machine uses magnetic waves to generate a detailed picture of the body's internal structures.

Medial collateral ligament (MCL) The ligament attaching the femur to the tibia, which is found outside the knee on the inner (medial) side of the leg.

Meniscus A half-moon-shaped cushion inside the knee, which acts as a shock absorber between the femur and tibia.

Microfracture An arthroscopic surgery procedure designed to repair articular cartilage by making tiny fractures of the bone where it meets the cartilage, creating an environment in which cartilage may grow.

Mosaicplasty A surgical procedure in which small, cylindrical pieces of bone with attached cartilage are packed together to restore cartilage surface.

MRI *See* Magnetic resonance imaging.

Naturopathy A therapy that relies on natural remedies, such as herbs, massage, and sunlight, to promote healing.

Nonsteroidal anti-inflammatory drugs (NSAIDs) A class of drugs used to reduce inflammation; it includes ibuprofen, Motrin, aspirin, Naprosyn, Dapro, Celebrex, Vioxx, and a multitude of others.

NSAIDs *See* Nonsteroidal anti-inflammatory drugs.

OKC exercises *See* Open kinetic chain exercises.

Open kinetic chain (OKC) exercises Exercises in which the foot is free to move; examples are leg lifts and curls.

Orthotics Mechanical devices, such as arch supports, designed to correct irregularities in gait, reduce pain, and reduce overuse injuries.

Osgood-Schlatter disease A painful syndrome of the lower knee that most commonly affects adolescent males; it is caused by repetitive stress or tension on the upper tibia where the patellar tendon inserts.

Osteoarthritis (degenerative arthritis) A condition in which the bone and cartilage in a joint break down; the most common form of arthritis, osteoarthritis may result simply from aging or may be triggered by injury or overuse.

Osteoblasts The cells that grow bone and make it dense.

Osteochondritis dessicans: A condition in which a portion of articular cartilage and underlying bone separates from the bone. Most common in the medial femoral condyle.

Osteoporosis A disease, more common in women than men, in which the bones become extremely porous; the lack of bone density greatly increases vulnerability to fracture, spinal deformity, and inhibited mobility.

Patella (kneecap) A flat, circular bone located at the front of the knee joint.

Patellofemoral syndrome (runner's knee) A condition in which the patella slips out of normal position, often because the tendon and supporting structures are either too loose or too tight, causing abrasion and inflammation; it usually occurs in reaction to the stress of repetitive movement.

Pathogen An agent, such as bacteria or viruses, that causes disease.

Plantar flexion Tilting of the foot downward at the ankle.

Plica Bands of synovial tissue that are left over from the earliest stages of fetal development and form a remnant pouch in a joint.

Plica syndrome Irritation and inflammation of the plica as a result of overuse or injury.

Posterior cruciate ligament (PCL) A ligament connecting the femur and the tibia, which is found inside and to the back of the knee joint.

Prolotherapy A pain-relieving injection therapy that promotes collagen growth in areas that have become inflamed or injured. *Prolo* refers to the proliferation of new cells.

Prostaglandin A substance produced by the body that protects the gastrointestinal tract from acid.

Q angle *See* Quadriceps angle.

Quadriceps The group of muscles in the front of the thigh.

Quadriceps angle (Q angle) The angle defined by a line drawn from the bump above and in front of the hip to the center the kneecap and a line from the kneecap to the tibial tuberosity.

Range of motion (ROM) The maximum amount that a particular joint can move; a knee whose movement is completely uninhibited is one with full ROM.

Rheumatoid arthritis A chronic form of arthritis believed to result from an autoimmune dysfunction in which the body has an immune response to its own cells or tissue.

RICE protocol A treatment consisting of rest, ice, compression, and elevation.

ROM *See* Range of motion.

Septic arthritis *See* Infectious arthritis.

Suturing Stitching together surgically.

Synovial tissue A thin tissue that lines many joints and produces a lubricating fluid.

Tai chi (tai chi chuan) An ancient Chinese exercise designed to promote strength, balance, mobility, and relaxation.

Tendinitis Inflammation of a tendon.

Tendon A band of tough, fibrous tissue that connects muscle to bone.

Thrombus A clot of blood in a blood vessel.

Tibia The larger, inner bone of the lower leg.

Valgus deformity A condition in which the knees are improperly aligned inward, such as knock-knees.

Valgus stress Pressure or an impact that forces the knee inward; when traumatic, it is a cause of ligament and meniscus injury.

Vastus medialis oblique (VMO) The inner or medial quadriceps muscle, which is primarily charged with keeping the patella from slipping laterally. A lax VMO may contribute to patellofemoral syndrome.

VMO *See* Vastus medialis oblique.

References

BROTZMAN, S. BRENT. *Clinical Orthopedic Rehabilitation*. St. Louis: Mosby, 1995.

BROWN, DAVID E., M.D., and RANDALL D. NEUMANN, M.D. *Orthopedic Secrets*. Philadelphia: Hanley and Belfus, Inc., 1995.

BURTON GOLDBERG GROUP, compiler. *Alternative Medicine: The Definitive Guide*. Fife, Wash.: Future Medicine Publishing, Inc., 1994.

EADES, MICHAEL R., M.D., and MARY DAN. *Protein Power*. New York: Bantam Books, 1998.

ETTINGER, WALTER H., JR., M.D., et al. "A Randomized Trial Comparing Aerobic Exercise and Resistance Exercise with a Health Education Program in Older Adults with Knee Osteoarthritis: The Fitness Arthritis and Seniors Trial (FAST)." *Journal of the American Medical Association* 277(1) (January 1, 1997): 25–31.

HAUSER, ROSS A., M.D. *Prolo Your Pain Away: Curing Chronic Pain with Prolotherapy*. Oak Park, Ill: Beulah Land Press, 1998.

HELMS, JOSEPH. *Medical Acupuncture Energetics: A Clinical Approach for Physicians*, illustrated by Glen McKenzie. Berkeley, Calif.: Medical Acupuncture Publishers, 1995.

HOPPENFELD, STANLEY, M.D. *Physical Examination of the Spine and Extremities*. Norwalk, Conn.: Appleton and Lange, 1976.

KLAPPER, ROBERT, M.D., and LYNDA HUEY. *Heal Your Hips: How to Prevent Hip Surgery—and What to Do If You Need It*. New York: John Wiley and Sons, 1999.

KUSTER, M. S., et al. "Endurance Sports After Total Knee Replacement: A Biochemical Investigation." *Medicine and Science in Sports and Exercise* 32(4) (April 2000): 721–724.

LIU, S. H., et al. "Estrogen Affects the Cellular Metabolism of the Anterior Cruciate Ligament: A Potential Explanation for Female Athletic Injury." *American Journal of Sports Medicine* 25(5) (September–October 1997): 704–709.

MAGEE, DAVID J., Ph.D., B.P.T. *Orthopedic Physical Assessment.* Philadelphia: W. B. Saunders Co., 1992.

MELLION, MORRIS B., M.D. *Sports Medicine Secrets.* Philadelphia: Hanley and Belfus, Inc., 1994.

Merck's 1899 Manual. New York: Merck and Co., 1899.

THEODOSAKIS, JASON, BARRY FOX, and BRENDA ADDERLY. *The Arthritis Cure: The Medical Miracle that Can Halt, Reverse, and May Even Cure Osteoarthritis.* New York: St. Martin's Press, 1997.

WEINSTOCK, RON J. "Magnetic Resonance Analyzer—A New Ray of Hope." *Physical Therapy Products*, July–August 1997, 76–78.

WOJTYS, E. M., et al. "Association Between the Menstrual Cycle and Anterior Cruciate Ligament Injuries in Female Athletes." *American Journal of Sports Medicine* 26(5) (September–October 1998): 614–619.

Index